USDA nutrition guidelines
http://www.mypyramid.gov

DATE DUE

~~OE 18 99~~			
~~OE~~			
~~MY 16 05~~			
~~DE 16 06~~			
EE 7 1 '10			

Dale Seymour Publications

White Plains, New York

...eymour Publications®, an imprint of Addison Wesley Longman, Inc.

...ns

White Plains, NY 10602
Customer Service: 800-872-1100

Funded under a grant from the United States Department of Agriculture, Nutrition Education and Training Program, in cooperation with Instructional Services, North Carolina Department of Public Instruction.

Senior Editor: Lois Fowkes
Design Manager: Jeff Kelly
Production Coordinator: Claire Flaherty
Production and cover illustration: Graham Metcalfe
Cover and text design: Paula Shuhert
Illustrations: Joel Snyder

Cheerios is a registered trademark of General Mills, Inc.
Cream of Wheat is a registered trademark of Nabisco, Inc.

ISBN 0-201-49452-3

DSP 49452

3 4 5 6 7-ML-02 01 00 99 98

Contents

Acknowledgments

This project was made possible by many individuals who provided support, guidance, and assistance.

Funding for the project was provided by the Healthful Living Section, North Carolina Department of Public Education. Linda Greene Hedquist, Project Coordinator for the North Carolina Department of Public Education, recognized the need for this resource, was instrumental in making the project possible, played a major role in the conceptualization stages of the work, and provided input and support throughout.

Nutritionists MaryAnn C. Farthing and Kim Dove provided in-depth consultation to project staff and helped to create the necessary link between the fields of early childhood education and nutrition, so that the required collaboration could take place.

The Advisory Board, listed below, is a knowledgeable group of expert reviewers who provided timely feedback on the materials and offered excellent suggestions.

Dr. Beverly Bryant
Department of Home Economics
North Carolina Central University

Jean Carter
Even Start
Department of Public Instruction

Katie Causon
Child Resources Center
Charlotte, North Carolina

Carolyn Dunn
North Carolina State University
Cooperative Extension Service
Home Economics

Georgia Enright
Rockingham Community College

Ray Hawkins
Child Nutrition Services
Department of Public Instruction

Vicki Lipscomb
Child Nutrition Program, Inc.
Charlotte, North Carolina

Jeanne Marlowe
Program Development Unit
Division of Child Development

Martha Myers
Child and Adult Care Feeding Program
Northwest Technical Assistance Center

Lucy Roberts
Early Childhood
Department of Public Instruction

Peggy Teague
Guilford Technical Community College
Jamestown Campus

Mary Thompson
Chapel Hill Carrboro Head Start

Betsy Thigpen
North Carolina Head Start Association

Pat Wesley
Frank Porter Graham Child Development Center

Patsy West
Southwest Technical Assistance Center

Pamela Rolandelli, a project staff member, reviewed all nutrition activities and provided many helpful ideas for improvements. In addition, she organized the tryout of many activities in preschool programs, during which we were able to observe the success of activities that appear in the book.

Isabelle Lewis, colleague and friend, reviewed the first draft of the manuscript and provided us with many activity ideas based on her experiences working with preschoolers over many years.

Activities were tested in several types of preschool programs, including child care, Head Start/public school preschool, and public school kindergarten. We wish to thank the many teachers and children in Chapel Hill-Carrboro Head Start, the Frank Porter Graham Child Development Center, Glenwood Elementary School, and Sycamore Preschoool, who tried the activities with us.

Cathy Riley took major responsibility for the word processing of the book, and was assisted by Hugh Siegel.

We are extremely thankful to all who contributed their interest, ideas, and support to make this work possible.

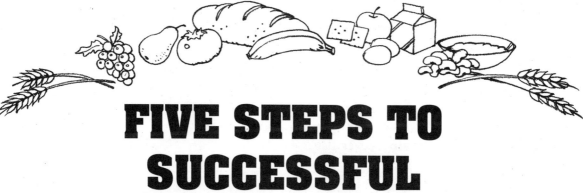

FIVE STEPS TO SUCCESSFUL NUTRITION EDUCATION

Five Steps to Successful Nutrition Education

Nutrition education for preschool-aged children needs to happen every day if it is to be successful. Nutrition education as a special, *sometimes* activity just does not get the message across. A consistent message that is a part of the children's everyday life in the early childhood program must be presented. Here are five major steps that can be taken to make nutrition education really work with preschoolers.

1 Serve healthful foods.

2 Provide pleasant meal and snack times.

3 Work with parents to encourage healthful eating habits.

4 Be a model of healthful eating for the children.

5 Make nutrition activities part of the daily learning environment.

Step 1
Serve Healthful Foods

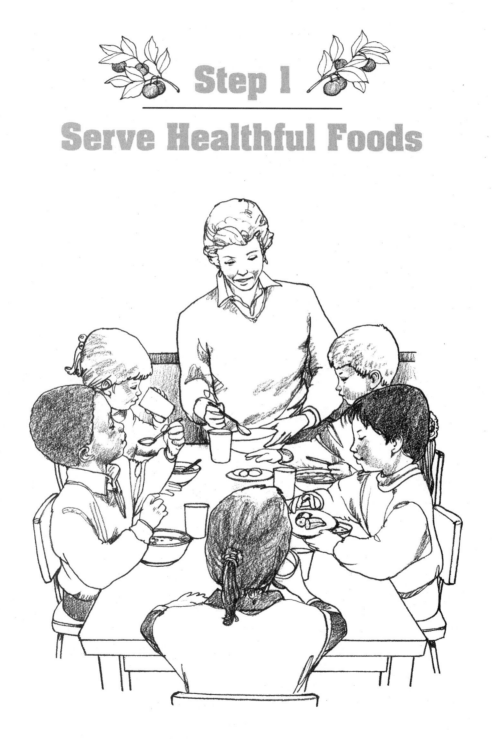

20 Nutrition Facts to Think About

As a teacher, you have the wonderful chance to help children grow to become strong, healthy, and competent. Children's nutrition is important to their health today and for the rest of their lives. Nutrition also makes a difference in how well children can learn.

You can do children a lifelong favor by reading these Nutrition Facts and then making sure the information is put into practice in your early childhood program every day. Throughout this book, these facts are explained more fully, with lots of ideas for using the information presented.

• • • • • • • Meeting Children's Health Needs • • • • • • •

 The foods served in programs for preschool-aged children are very important for the nutritional health of the child. Eating well at home will not make up for what preschoolers might miss during the day.

 When there is too little variety in the foods children eat, it is difficult to meet their nutritional needs.

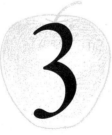 Eating too much food over time with too little activity may cause children to become overweight.

 Eating too many foods that contain a lot of fat may lead to health problems later in life.

 Many preschoolers, especially those from low-income families, are at risk for iron-deficiency anemia.

 Iron, vitamin A, B-vitamins, calcium, and vitamin C are sometimes deficient in the total amount of food eaten by preschoolers, especially those from low-income families.

 Eating sweet, sticky foods too often can lead to tooth decay, especially if proper dental hygiene such as tooth brushing does not follow eating these foods.

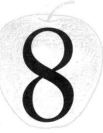 Poorly nourished children do not learn as well as children who eat plenty of healthful foods.

Respecting Children's Food Choices

A child's dislike of a food should be respected, just as an adult's is.

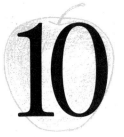
Preschoolers dislike cooked vegetables, especially those that taste bitter, more than any other food. Some children dislike meats, especially if they are hard to chew. Trying different vegetables prepared in different ways will often increase the child's eating of vegetables. When a child dislikes a food, another food of similar value should be substituted if possible.

Rewards and punishments should never be used to encourage children to eat.

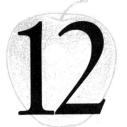
All of the people involved in a child's eating experiences influence the child's eating habits. This includes parents, family members, friends, teachers, and others. When these influential people choose to eat healthful foods, children are more likely to do the same.

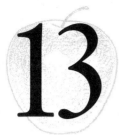 Children know best how much they want to eat. Suggested serving amounts of foods will meet the needs of the average child, but no child should ever be forced to eat these amounts.

 Preschoolers may not always want to try a new food the first time it is served to them. No fuss should be made if the child does not like a food; just try again once in a while.

Encouraging Children to Enjoy Healthful Foods

 Children are more likely to accept a new food when they have learned about it before trying it.

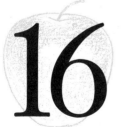 Children grow faster at some ages than at others. Three- to five-year-olds usually grow slowly, so they may not be as interested in eating as they were when they were babies.

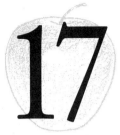

17 Teachers and parents should work together to encourage good eating habits at home and in the early childhood program and share what they know about the healthful foods the child will or will not eat.

18 Meals served to the children should be attractive, or have *child appeal*. Textures should be chewy, soft, or crisp—not tough. Flavors should be mild and neither too salty nor too spicy. Temperatures should not be too cold nor too hot. Colors should be bright. Serving sizes should fit the child's need.

19 Mealtimes should be happy times with little stress and confusion. If healthful meals with child appeal are served in a pleasant setting with child-sized tables, chairs, dishes, and utensils, then children will be more likely to enjoy the foods and eat what they need.

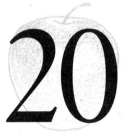

20 Children should be able to eat in a matter-of-fact way, with sufficient amounts of foods to meet their health needs. Meal and snack times should be made no more and no less important than other activities of the day.

Have a dependable meal and snack schedule

Preschoolers get grumpy, have more fights, and do not learn well when they are hungry, so it's important to be sure that children do not have to wait too long for meals and snacks. Eating times should be evenly spaced through the day and should occur at about the same time from day to day. A good meal/snack schedule that works well for preschoolers should look like this:

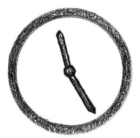

Preschoolers' Meal and Snack Schedule

Early Morning:	➡	Breakfast
Mid-morning:	➡	Snack
Noon:	➡	Lunch
Mid-afternoon:	➡	Snack
Early Evening:	➡	Dinner
Before Bedtime:	➡	Snack

The number of meals and snacks children are served in their preschool program should depend on how long they attend each day. What children eat at home cannot make up for what they might miss while they are in the program.

Sometimes your program's meal/snack schedule may need to be modified to meet a child's special requirements. For example, if you notice that a child comes to your program hungry every morning and the parent has not responded to your breakfast suggestions, you might want to consider serving an earlier morning snack. The schedule may also need changes to meet the special needs of a child with a disability. For example, a child who has difficulty digesting food may need to be served smaller meals or snacks more often than other children.

Serve healthful foods at meals and snacks

Some preschoolers are growing quickly while others may be growing more slowly. All preschoolers use lots of energy as they play and learn, so they need plenty of nutritious foods to help them grow strong and healthy. Since preschoolers have small stomachs, they are not able to eat large amounts of food at one time. They do better when offered smaller amounts of food more frequently. That's why both healthful meals *and snacks* are necessary to meet children's nutritional needs.

Serve a variety of healthful foods

Almost every child will like or dislike certain foods. Some children are more willing than others to try new foods. To be sure that children eat to meet their nutritional needs, serve a variety of healthful foods. Then children will have lots of good choices to enjoy. The more different foods a child tries, the more likely the child will be to eat everything that's needed for good nutrition.

To ensure variety, remember the food groups

To be sure children get the variety of foods they need every day, it helps to think about the food groups used to classify different foods. Make sure that foods from each group are served every day. These food groups are based on the nutrients they contribute to the total diet.

Food Groups

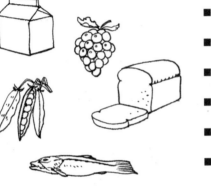

- Bread, Cereal, Rice, and Pasta Group

- Vegetable Group

- Fruit Group

- Milk, Yogurt, and Cheese Group

- Meat, Poultry, Fish, Dry Beans, Eggs, and Nuts Group

- Fats, Oils, and Sweets Group

Use the Food Guide Pyramid

The United States Department of Agriculture (USDA) has provided an easy way to remember how much of each food group people need every day for healthful eating. The Food Guide Pyramid shows clearly which foods should be eaten more often and which should be eaten less often.

A Guide to Daily Food Choices

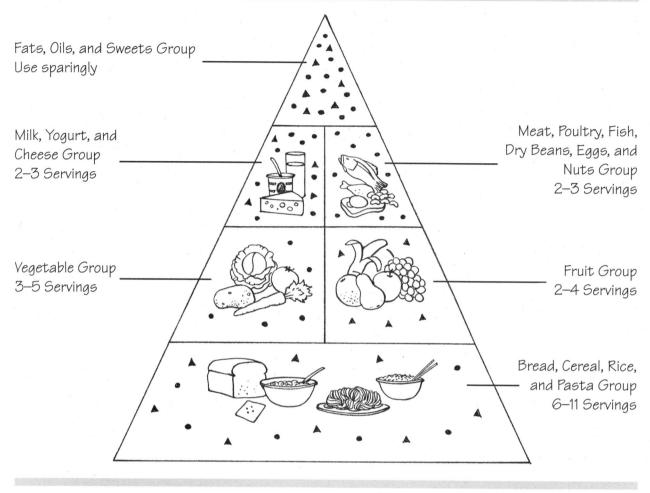

Fats, Oils, and Sweets Group
Use sparingly

Milk, Yogurt, and
Cheese Group
2–3 Servings

Meat, Poultry, Fish,
Dry Beans, Eggs, and
Nuts Group
2–3 Servings

Vegetable Group
3–5 Servings

Fruit Group
2–4 Servings

Bread, Cereal, Rice,
and Pasta Group
6–11 Servings

KEY

● Fat (naturally occurring and added)

▲ Sugars (added)

These symbols show naturally occurring and added fat and sugar in foods.

Serve small amounts and allow seconds

Children usually do not eat very much at one time, but sometimes they may surprise you and eat lots of one thing they really enjoy. This is fine, as long as everything they can choose from is healthful. You will find that a child's appetite is greater when the child is going through a growth spurt or has just recovered from an illness.

Large amounts on a plate can discourage a child, so give small servings to each child. Be sure to have extra food and drink available for children who want seconds. The USDA Child and Adult Food Program requires that meals and snacks served in a preschool program include minimum amounts shown in the chart.

Suggested Servings for Preschoolers

Breakfast

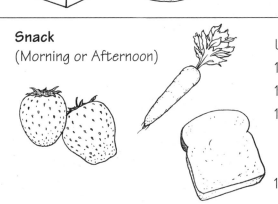

1/2 cup fruit or juice or vegetable

1/2 slice bread

   or 1/3 cup cold cereal

   or 1/4 cup cooked cereal

3/4 cup fluid milk* (whole or 2%)

Snack
(Morning or Afternoon)

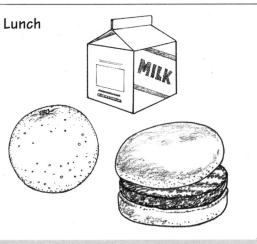

Use two choices at each snack:

1/2 ounce meat or meat alternative

1/2 cup fruit or juice or vegetable

1/2 slice bread

   or 1/3 cup dry cereal

   or 1/4 cup cooked cereal

1/2 cup fluid milk* (whole or 2%)

Lunch

1-1/2 ounces cooked meat, poultry, or fish

   or 1-1/2 ounces cheese

   or 1 egg

   or 2/3 cup dry beans/peas

   or 3 tablespoons peanut butter**

1/2 cup vegetable or fruit

1/2 slice bread or bread alternative, such as cornbread, muffin, rice, macaroni

3/4 cup fluid milk* (whole or 2%)

*   Milk must be fluid milk. Powdered milk, skim milk, yogurt, cheese, and other milk products should not be substituted for the fluid milk.

**   One tablespoon of peanut butter on a small sandwich will not meet this requirement.

Source: United States Department of Agriculture

Never force children to eat or allow a child to go hungry

Children, like adults, come in many different sizes. Each child will have a different appetite, so it's important to remember that each child knows best how much he or she wants to eat. Suggested serving sizes will meet the nutrition needs of the average child, but these guidelines should never be used to force an amount of food on any child or to make a child go hungry. Unless the child's physician instructs otherwise, children should be allowed to eat healthful foods until they feel satisfied. If a child's parents request that the child's eating be limited, ask for a note from the child's doctor listing restrictions that you should follow.

Never force children to eat foods they dislike

Preschoolers will usually tell you very clearly what they like and do not like to eat. A child's dislike of a food should be respected, just as an adult's is. It is easier and quicker to change the food than to change the child.

Try several times and in several different ways to introduce a new food to a child. It's possible that the child will develop a taste for a new food over time, but keep in mind that most adults like certain foods more than others.

Sometimes preschoolers go on food jags and want to eat only a very limited number of foods. For example, some preschoolers may want to eat peanut butter sandwiches and little else. This is usually a temporary behavior, although to the adult it may seem endless, and children usually seem to focus on relatively healthful foods.

To be sure that a child gets the nutrition needed for growth and good health, it is best to go along with food preferences while continuing to add a variety of foods to each meal and snack. In an early childhood program, the child will probably be offered the needed variety of foods at meals and snacks. When the child is at home, the parents are more likely to allow the child to eat the preferred foods, but they should also try to encourage greater variety in the child's diet.

Encourage children to try a new food by teaching them about it

You can help children to be more accepting of a new food when you teach them something about it before they try it. Talking or reading a book about where the food comes from, how it helps children to grow strong and be well, and how it is prepared are some ways to get children interested in a food before the first taste. Allowing children to help prepare the food is even more rewarding. Children are much more likely to eat foods that they have fixed themselves. Many ideas that make trying new foods fun are provided in the Nutrition Activities section.

Replace foods not liked with other foods having the same value

If children dislike a food that is served for a meal or snack, it is best to simply offer a different food of equal value the next time. As long as you replace a healthful food with another similar healthful food, you will not decrease the nutritional value. For example, if cooked carrots are served at lunch and almost no one eats them, then raw carrots, cut into strips, or another raw or cooked vegetable that the children do like should be offered. Any foods that the children do not enjoy can be tried from time to time, but they should not be served frequently or all together. This will help ensure that the children get the foods they need to grow strong and healthy.

You will find a list of foods that can be substituted for other foods in Appendix A.

When children's dislikes are respected and other foods are substituted, then mealtimes are less likely to turn into frustrating battles. Children's tastes will change as they get older, and they will usually learn to enjoy more and more foods. The important things to remember are to keep mealtimes pleasant and offer healthful foods to children.

Remember

Keep mealtimes pleasant.

Offer healthful foods to children.

Be sure to meet any special nutrition needs

Some children may have special nutritional needs that must be met for the child's healthy growth. For example, a child who is allergic to milk must be provided with a milk substitute when milk is served, and adults must be aware of the allergy so that the child does not eat any foods that might cause an allergic reaction. A list of all children's allergies should be posted where adults can easily see it so that no child is ever served foods that cause health problems.

Most children with disabilities will not differ from typically developing children in what they eat or in how they are fed. They will want to learn how to feed themselves, clean up, and enjoy eating with friends just as everyone else does. As with all children, it is best to check with the child's parents when the child is enrolled to determine abilities and find out about preferences. Then you can work with the child and family members to help establish healthful eating habits.

Some children with disabilities may have special feeding requirements. For example, a child with a motor disability may find it difficult to chew or control a spoon and require some extra help from you. Another child may have a medical condition that makes digesting food difficult and may require special feeding. The food preparation person in your program may need to prepare foods in a special way so that the child can eat them more easily. You will want to cooperate with the child's parents and the professionals who are working with the child—the physical therapist, nutritionist or registered dietitian, occupational therapist, speech-language pathologist— to make any special arrangements that are needed for proper feeding.

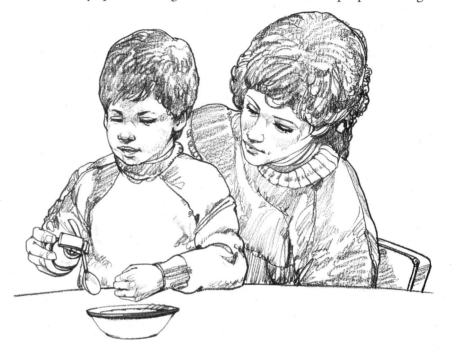

Serve meals with child appeal

Children are more likely to eat well when meals look and taste good to them. Here are some tips to remember that make children more eager to eat the foods served:

- Food textures should be chewy, soft, or crisp—not tough.
- Flavors should be mild—many preschoolers do not like strong flavors.
- Foods should not be too hot or too cold.
- Colors of foods should be bright.
- Serving sizes should fit the child's appetite.

Communicate with cooks to help provide meals with child appeal

Teachers who supervise meals and snacks really know which foods the children enjoy and which ones they just will not eat. Many programs have cooks who prepare meals and snacks for the children. Other programs receive meals from off-site kitchens, such as public school cafeterias or community kitchens. To ensure that children eat the foods that are prepared for them, it is up to the teacher to communicate with the cooking staff about how children respond to the foods they are being served.

The good teacher will communicate with the cook or menu planner to talk about the foods that the children will not eat and to suggest other nutritious substitutes. For example, many preschoolers do not like chicken noodle casserole because they simply dislike foods that are all mixed up. The teacher might suggest that the noodles, vegetables, and chicken be served separately instead of as a casserole, so that the children are more likely to eat the meal.

Limit sugar and fats

The foods served to children should help rather than hinder the child's healthy growth. If preschoolers fill up on foods that are low in nutrients, such as most cookies, chips, sugary drinks, or even too much juice, then there will be little room left in their stomachs for the foods that are nutritious. To give children the best chance for good health, offer plenty of the nutritious foods and only small amounts of foods that are low in nutrients.

Eating too many foods that are high in sugar and fat is also related to weight problems. Severe health risks throughout life are related to excess weight and fat intake.

Sweet, sticky foods can cause tooth decay

Although children may like sugary foods, you are not doing children a favor when you often give them sweets to eat. Eating too many foods that are sweet can cause tooth decay. Tooth decay is painful, costly when treated, and may lead to the loss of permanent teeth. The effects of sugar on the teeth can be reduced by proper brushing after eating sweets. If sweets are served in the early childhood program, tooth brushing should always follow.

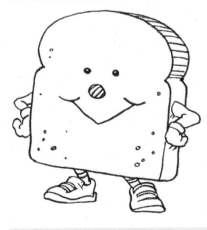

Do Children a Favor

Limit		Serve Instead
Candy, cookies	⇒	Fruits, graham crackers
Soft drinks, sugary drinks	⇒	100% fruit juice, milk
Cakes, doughnuts	⇒	Fruit muffins and breads with low fat content
Sugar-coated cereals	⇒	Plain cereals with fruit

Too many fatty foods may cause health problems later in life

Foods that are high in fat are unfortunately just as popular as sweets. French fries, fried chicken and fried fish, potato chips, sausage, cheese, and cream are just a few examples of these high-fat foods. Fat from animal sources such as fatty meats, butter, and lard is related to risks of clogged arteries, which may cause heart disease and high blood pressure later in life. In addition, all fatty foods are high in calories and may cause problems with gaining too much weight in later years.

Even though children may like fatty foods because they find them tasty, these foods should be limited. They take up space in the child's small stomach so that the child will not be hungry for more nutritious foods.

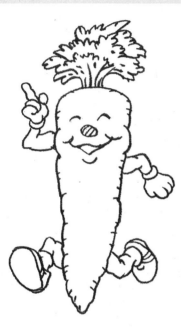

Do Children a Favor

Limit	Serve Instead
Cookies, doughnuts, cakes	Cereals, breads, fruits
Vegetables cooked with fatback	Crisp-cooked or raw vegetables
Deep- or pan-fried foods	Broiled, baked or boiled foods
Fatty meats, such as bologna, sausage, bacon and hot dogs	Skinless chicken and turkey; fish, eggs, lean meats including lean beef and lean pork
Ice cream	Fruit juice bars

Lower the chances of iron-deficiency anemia with a variety of healthful foods

Preschoolers, especially those from low-income families, are at risk for iron-deficiency anemia. Iron-deficiency anemia causes children to be tired, less active than others, and unable to learn well. Children with this problem may also grow slowly. When a variety of healthful foods is served each day, children are less likely to suffer from iron-deficiency anemia. Serving foods that are high in iron is very important. Eating a variety of healthful foods makes it more likely that a child will get enough iron and other nutrients needed to avoid anemia.

Do Children a Favor

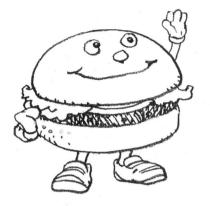

Serve Foods High in Iron

- Lean meat
- Enriched and whole grain breads and cereals
- Cream of Wheat®
- Dried fruit (peaches, prunes, apricots, raisins)
- Dried beans (pinto, navy, kidney)
- Greens (collard, kale, mustard, spinach, turnip greens)

Preschoolers get other important vitamins and minerals from a variety of foods

Besides iron, there is sometimes not enough vitamin A, vitamin C, B-vitamins, and calcium in the total amount of food eaten by preschoolers. All of these are needed for healthy bodies.

Vitamin A is needed for healthy skin, good vision, and growth. Vitamin C is needed for healthy gums. Children will get these vitamins if they eat plenty of fruits and vegetables.

B-vitamins are usually found in enriched breakfast cereals and enriched breads. Whole grain foods, such as whole-wheat bread or oatmeal, also contain B-vitamins. These are needed to help our bodies grow normally.

Calcium helps build strong bones and teeth. Milk and milk products such as yogurt, cheese, and cottage cheese supply calcium, as do products made from soybeans, such as tofu.

Snacks should be healthful mini-meals

Some people are surprised to learn that it is a good idea to serve snacks to preschoolers. They think of snacks as unhealthful foods like soda, candy, and chips that keep children from eating well at mealtimes. But in a good preschool program, snacks are nutritious little meals that allow children to refuel until mealtime. The snack foods served in good programs are as nutritious as the foods served at meals. Since preschoolers cannot eat much at one time, healthful snacks help ensure that children eat enough recommended foods throughout the day to meet their nutritional needs.

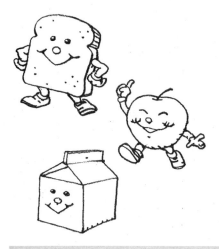

Healthful Snacks Are

- Made up of a variety of healthful foods and drinks

- Made up of the same types of healthful foods that are served at meals

- Small servings that don't make the child too full to eat at mealtime

- Often easy for children to prepare

- A good way to add variety to all the foods eaten in a day

Make sure foods are not choking hazards

Preschoolers are more likely to choke on foods than older children. Their throats are smaller and they do not chew thoroughly. The foods that have caused most deaths from choking include hot dogs, nuts, hard candies, and grapes. Here are some easy steps to take to minimize the risk of choking.

- Supervise children carefully during meals and snacks.

- Do not allow children to play or walk or run around while eating. Activity makes supervision of eating more difficult and increases the chances of choking.

- Try not to hurry children who are eating.

- Serve a drink with all meals and snacks so that children can take a sip to wash down dry foods as they eat. Do not wait until after the children have finished eating to serve the drink.

- Encourage small bites and lots of chewing.

- Gently remind children to talk only after they have swallowed.

- Serve foods in small pieces. Cut up foods that might choke a child. Narrow strips are less likely to cause choking than chunks.

- Avoid serving hard candies and popcorn to children who are three years or younger. Hot dogs can be served if cut into narrow strips (not round slices). Nuts must be chopped into small pieces. Grapes should be cut into quarters. Hard fruits and vegetables should be shredded, grated, or cut into narrow strips. Peanut butter should be spread very thinly.

- Take extra care with a child who has a disability that increases chances of choking. Be sure to consistently carry out all precautions suggested by the child's parents and the specialists who work with the child.

Serve healthful party foods

Lots of sweets and fatty foods are often served at parties and celebrations. Children learn to think that these foods are special and better than the healthful foods they usually eat. This should not happen. Children should learn that parties are fun when healthful foods are combined with special activities for children to enjoy. For example, children can plan their own menus for a special day and then prepare the foods themselves. Or they can decorate tables with placemats and a table centerpiece they make. There are many ideas for healthful party foods in the Nutrition Activities section of this book.

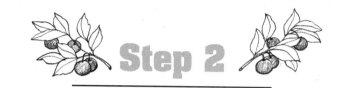

Step 2

Provide Pleasant Meal and Snack Times

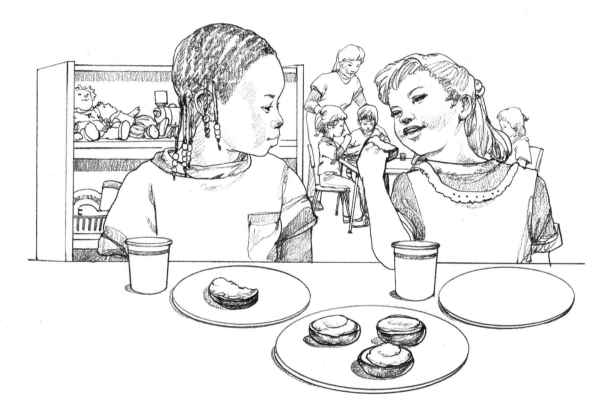

Meal and snack times should be pleasant social times

Meal and snack times should be relaxed and pleasant for children and adults. Forcing children to eat foods they do not like or controlling their behavior through harsh methods may lead to lifelong eating problems. Insuring pleasant eating times with groups of preschoolers takes thoughtful planning and organization. When planning eating experiences, it helps to think about what should happen before eating, while eating, and after eating.

Pre-meal activities should calm children and minimize waiting

Allow preschoolers to be busily involved in interesting activities before meals. Long waiting times with nothing to do cause children to become restless and to behave badly. Then adults and children are stressed, and the chance for a pleasant meal or snack is lost.

Keeping children in one large group also causes problems. Young children do not handle large groups very well. They do far better in small groups or just playing with a friend. To ease children into a meal or snack time, plan before-meal activities that do not require children to wait or to be in one large, crowded group. Here are some ideas for moving children into eating times smoothly:

- Allow a few children to set tables, or have individuals take turns setting their places while others are doing other activities.

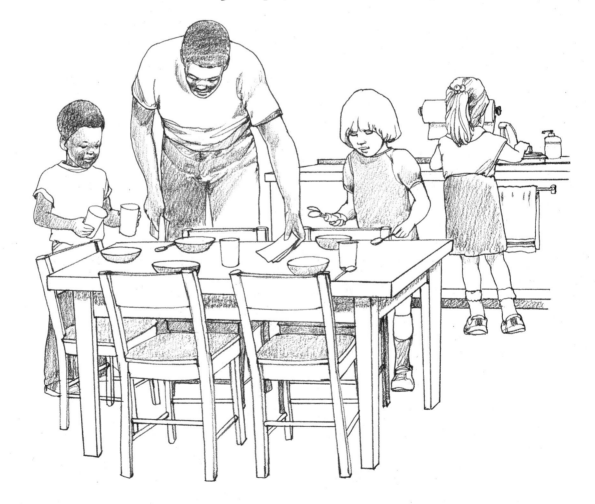

Five Steps to Successful Nutrition Education

- Allow children to play and be actively involved until food is already on the table. Children should not be expected to eat immediately following very active play. Before sitting down to eat, a short period of quiet play, such as listening to a story or singing, should be scheduled for those who are not washing hands or helping with meal preparation. Then children will not be too keyed up to eat.

- Send a few children to wash hands at a time so that there will be less waiting and crowding.

- Have children sit down at the table only when food is already served so that children won't have to wait with nothing to do.

Plan and set up a good mealtime area

Meals and snacks are most pleasant when children can learn to do things for themselves and are free to socialize with friends. Good planning is needed to ensure that meals are happy and problem free.

The first thing to plan is a good physical setting for the eating experience. For pleasant meals, the following things should be provided in the early childhood setting:

- Safe, easy-to-use, and easily cleaned child-sized chairs and tables

- Floors that are easy to clean

- Child-sized pitchers, plates, cups, serving spoons, and eating utensils

- A convenient place to wash hands

Help children learn to be independent and competent

One of the most valuable gifts good teachers give to children is a sense of competence and independence. Meals and snacks are perfect times to help children learn to do things for themselves. There are many things that preschoolers can learn to do on their own. Patient teaching will pay off in the end.

Teach children to minimize the spread of germs

Making sure that germs are not spread at mealtimes is very important for the health of both children and adults. Of course, teachers will have to take much of the responsibility for sanitary procedures during meals and snacks. They must ensure that tables are sanitized properly; clean plates, cups, and utensils are used; and that food is served at the proper temperatures. But children can learn to take an active part in sanitary procedures, too.

Proper hand washing is one of the ways to avoid the spread of germs. Children can easily be taught to wash their hands before meals and after going to the bathroom. They need to be able to reach the water, soap, and towels safely and easily. Provide a low sink or a sink with a sturdy skid-proof step stool, and put soap and individual towels within the children's reach. Children should be reminded to wash hands before eating meals and snacks and before helping to prepare foods or setting the table.

Children can also learn to eat only the food served to them on their own plates. Adults must supervise carefully to be sure that children do not forget the boundaries and reach onto another child's plate or eat with a shared spoon. Boundaries are clear to adults, but it takes longer for children to realize that these limits are important.

Provide child-sized furnishings and equipment

Using child-sized furniture helps children feel competent while eating. They do not have to depend on an adult to push them up to the table; their feet can reach the floor. Child-sized tables and chairs allow children to sit comfortably with their feet on the floor, the table top within easy reach. Also, they feel more secure because they do not have to worry about falling from chairs, kneeling on chairs, or having their feet dangle. Tables that are the right height also permit children to see the food on their plate.

Special chairs or other equipment for children with certain disabilities may be needed so that all children, including those with disabilities, can eat with friends. Sometimes it will take special planning with the professionals who work with the child to be sure the necessary furniture is in place. But the time will be well spent if you ensure that a child with a disability can eat meals and snacks with a friendly group of children.

Spoons, forks, plates, and cups should be unbreakable so that children are safe while they learn how to use these items properly. They should also be child-sized so that children can manage by themselves. Child-sized utensils and equipment help children feel in control of their actions.

Children with disabilities may need specially adapted equipment, such as cups with rocker bottoms, bowls with high sides, or spoons with curved handles, to make independent eating possible. The specialists working with the child will have suggestions to help the child grow toward independence. It is likely that you will get new ideas about the equipment the child needs in order to become competent in your work during meals and snacks. Be sure to talk about your ideas with the child's parents and specialists.

Teach children to serve themselves

Children can learn many self-help skills when meals are served family style. This means that foods are placed on the table in bowls and drinks are served from pitchers or other containers. These serving containers are passed around the table so that all children can take turns serving themselves. This might seem to be a lot of extra work at first, and it will depend on the type of foods you serve, but you will be amazed at how well your preschoolers can do and how much they enjoy serving themselves.

You can encourage competence and independence by setting up the serving to be easy for the children's small hands. To help children learn to pour milk and other drinks by themselves, beverages should be poured into small pitchers (such as a 2-cup plastic measuring cup) that are placed on the table. Then children can learn to fill their own cups and pass the pitcher to the next child. Small serving bowls and spoons can be used so that children can serve their own portions of food.

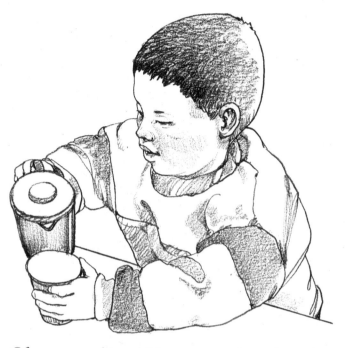

Of course, teaching children to serve themselves takes more involvement by the teacher, who must watch carefully at first. Children will need to be reminded to pass things to the next person, and a child with a disability might need a little extra help or reminding. But children soon learn to handle pouring milk and serving with great confidence. Your patient interest is rewarded with the knowledge that you have made it possible for children to learn new skills.

Spills always occur, so make it possible for children to clean up for themselves

It is difficult for preschoolers to eat without spilling food or drinks onto tables and floors. They just do not have the control needed to avoid spills. It's best to be ready for spills and use them as a learning time. Then no one will get upset when accidents happen.

Easy-to-clean floors in the eating area help both teachers and children do a better job with cleaning spills. Preschoolers feel competent when taught how to clean up their own spills properly. Small sponges, paper towels, a trash can, and a bucket with water should be nearby for this. Adults do children a favor when they are patient and teach children to clean spills up by themselves. This makes mealtimes more pleasant. Be sure children wash hands after cleaning up.

Encourage pleasant social times at the table

While learning to become competent and independent at meals, children can also learn how to cooperate and have relaxed conversations with each other. Pleasant mealtimes can be used to encourage positive social skills in children. To encourage positive social interaction at meal and snack times, it helps to remember these tips:

- Arrange for small groups of children to eat together. Have meals/snacks in the children's classroom rather than in one large cafeteria or dining room. Large rooms with many children lead to noisy mealtimes and tempt teachers to strictly enforce "No Talking" rules.

- Use smaller tables rather than one large table to limit the number of children and encourage quiet talk while eating. Be sure to include children with disabilities that require special equipment at the table so that all the children can eat in small social groups.

- Allow children to eat as soon as they are served.

- Allow children to leave the table and go to another activity when finished eating. Slow eaters should not be hurried but should be given plenty of time to finish.

- Have adults sit and eat with children. They can then act as models for how to behave.

- Encourage good manners gently—with quiet reminders and by setting a good example at all times.

- Do not make a big fuss about a child's misbehavior or lack of skills in handling food. No child should serve as an example of poor behavior. Upset children do not have happy food experiences.

Help children learn to have pleasant mealtime conversations

Use the following tips to help children have pleasant conversations during meals and snacks:

- Start conversations by asking questions about things that the children enjoyed doing during the day's activities. ("Tell us about the block supermarket you built this morning." . . . "How did you help to fix this salad?")

- Be sure to include all children in the conversations, including those who have disabilities. If a child uses signing or needs special equipment, such as a communication board, be sure that this is made a regular part of meals and snacks.

- Show the children how to act by setting a good example. Look and listen when a child speaks to you. Allow the child to take several turns talking so that the conversation is extended.

- Bring up topics that you think are interesting. See if the children join in and then help keep the conversation going.

- Serve as a referee and troubleshooter. If children are talking together, keep one ear open for signs of trouble.

- Make sure all children get a turn to talk if they want to. Gently help children take turns in the talk. ("I think Jesse wants to say something. You can chew and swallow while Jesse takes a turn.")

- Set limits if necessary. Change the subject if things become unpleasant. Remind children about using soft voices indoors.

- Gently remind children to eat if they seem to be forgetting. For example, "I think you'll enjoy your cornbread, Brenda. Try a little, and then we can talk some more."

Encourage good manners in an appropriate way

Good manners become a true part of children's eating behavior when they are learned gradually. The most effective way to teach good manners is by showing children how to act. This works much better than threatening, embarrassing, or punishing children for bad manners.

Children will not really learn good manners unless they see adults using good manners. It's true that they may behave well while an adult is acting as a police officer, but as soon as the adult leaves, everything will change. So it's best to be more patient and treat children like honored guests at meals and snacks. Then they will learn that politeness is for everyone.

Never use food as a punishment or reward

Since children need nutritious foods to grow strong and healthy, no foods should ever be withheld as a punishment. Preventing children from having the foods they need can compromise the health of a child. Since "desserts" should be just as healthful as other foods served, these foods should not be withheld or used as bribes to win children over. Since sugary and fatty snack foods should be limited, they should never be used as rewards. When any foods are used as rewards, children learn to value them more than other foods. This can lead to overeating, as children (and, later, adults) use food to comfort or reward themselves.

Make the time after eating go smoothly

As children finish eating, you can encourage them to become independent and competent in many other ways. Preschoolers are capable of clearing their places and moving on to the next activity when things are planned and set up to go smoothly. Here are some things to remember:

- Have a large trash can near the eating area so that children can easily throw away paper and plastic plates, cups, utensils, and napkins. You may also choose to use this trash can for foods and drinks that have not been consumed.

- If nondisposable items are used, teach the children where to put them. Dishes can be placed in large dishpans or stacked on a serving cart. You may choose another method, but if you notice that children do not easily learn what to do, think of an easier way.

- Have a clean sponge that fits children's small hands so that they can wipe off tables. Teach them how to do this—how to rinse the sponge, wring out the extra water, and wipe carefully before an adult completes the cleanup with disinfectant or antibacterial wash.

- To avoid hectic times after eating, make sure children are busy and supervised by an adult. Be sure children know the next activities they will go to after clearing their place. Trouble often starts when teachers are busy cleaning up and children are left alone with little supervision. If needed, postpone final cleanup of the eating area until children are settled into the next activity.

- Have children wash their hands and brush their teeth after meals and, if possible, after snacks, too. If only one sink is available, one or two children can brush at a time while others are involved in different activities. If children must wait for a teacher to supervise toothbrushing, have another quiet activity ready for them to do.

Check to be certain meals and snacks are going well

Providing pleasant meal and snack times is easier when you stand back a little and think about how those routines are working. A checklist can help you find out what you are already doing well. It will also let you see where you might make some improvements. The Mealtime Checklist, which you will find in Appendix J, is easy to use and will be helpful in planning improvements in your program.

Five Steps to Successful Nutrition Education

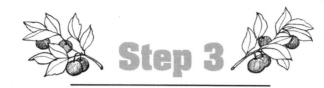

Step 3

Work with Parents to Encourage Healthful Eating Habits

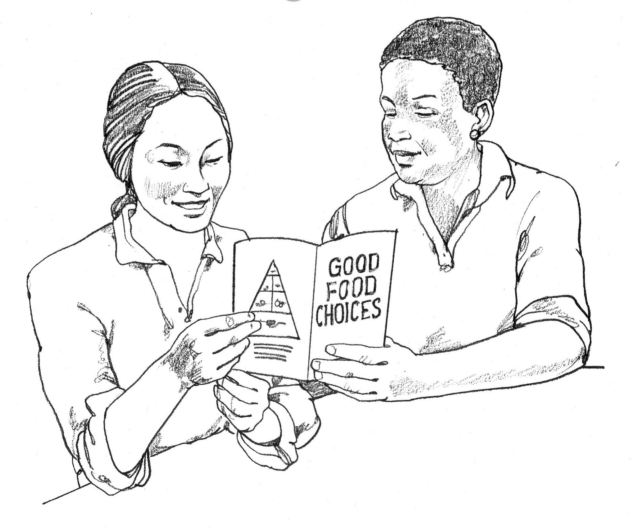

Work with parents to encourage healthful eating habits

Although you can have some influence on how and what children eat at school, parents usually have the greatest effect on a child's nutrition. That's why teachers and parents should work together to make sure the child has the best chance to learn to eat for good health.

You can help parents extend healthful eating into the home, and parents will have lots of good suggestions to share about foods their children enjoy. The ideas suggested below work well to bring teachers and parents together.

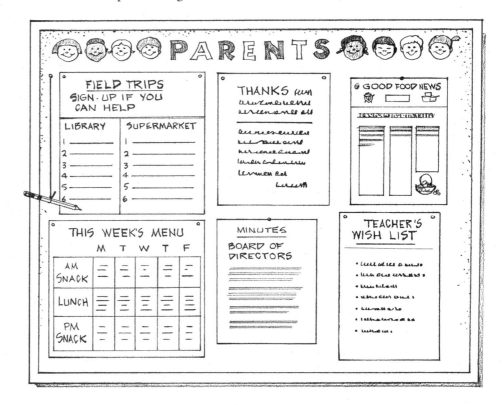

Help parents to understand your food program

- Display menus of all meals and snacks served each day and point them out to parents. Parents can then be sure their child gets a variety of foods by serving foods that are not listed on the daily menus. If possible, give a menu of all meals and snacks to each parent either weekly or monthly.

- Some local newspapers publish the menus for the public schools. If your early childhood program is part of the public schools, see if the menu for your program can also be printed.

- Encourage parents to eat lunch often with their children. This will enable them to see how meals are handled in their children's program and will add to the parent's and child's sense of closeness and belonging.

- During a conference with parents, discuss how meals and snacks are handled in your program. Encourage them to discuss with you the child's eating experience at home.

Engage in two-way communications about the child

- Make sure parents have told you about any foods the child cannot eat due to allergies or cultural, religious, or philosophical preferences related to foods. Post a list where you and other teachers can easily see it. Be sure that the child does not eat these foods and that another food of similar value is substituted.

- Give all parents a list of the healthful foods their child really enjoys. Have parents give you a list of the healthful foods the child eats at home. Then compare the lists. Try to figure out a way to serve home foods at the early childhood program and suggest that foods from the early childhood program be served at home.

Provide parents with basic nutrition information

- Display posters about healthful foods where parents are likely to see them. You will find some sources for posters in Appendix E, pages 189–190.

- Provide pamphlets about nutrition for parents to take home and read. You will find some sources for pamphlets in Appendix E.

- Have discussions about family nutrition and meal planning at parent meetings.

- Add articles on nutrition to your program's regular newsletter that is sent home to parents.

- Hand out nutrition newsletters, such as the ones for you to use that are included in Appendix B.

Encourage parents to bring in nutritious foods for children

- If parents provide snacks or lunches from home for their children, hand out newsletters or pamphlets with easy, healthful ideas. Ask that certain foods, such as chips or candy, not be brought to school.

- If parents take turns providing snacks for all the children in the group, then provide a list of healthful foods and drinks for parents to choose from. Help parents understand the importance of limiting foods that are high in sugar and fat.

- If parents wish to bring in foods for parties or other special occasions, be sure they know which foods are preferred in your classroom. Always avoid embarrassing parents who might bring in foods that are not your choice. You can guide parents by providing a list of suggestions. When the child is first enrolled, have parents sign up to bring in certain things from the list.

Include nutrition information in a resource center for parents

To give parents a chance to read nutrition information as well as general parenting advice, you may wish to set up a resource center for parents to use. This does not need to be costly or take lots of time. Staff and parents can work together to collect or make materials that can be available on loan for use by parents and children.

What to include

Since families will have different information needs, provide a wide variety of information in the resource center. Have some materials that do not require much time to use and others that give more detail. Include materials for children to look at while parents browse.

- Adult reading materials about human development (physical, social, emotional, and intellectual) covering the whole age range: prenatal, early and middle childhood, adolescence, adulthood, and old age.

- Information on parenting, children's nutritional and health needs, children's behavior, early learning, and activities for parents to share with children.

- Newspaper or magazine articles cut out and mounted in folders, materials collected in courses or workshops, pamphlets, bulletins, newsletters, magazines, and books.

- Materials for adults to use with children, such as children's books, activity boxes, toys, puzzles, and games. These can be parent- or teacher-made, donated, new, or used. Make sure that items are in reasonable condition. For example, puzzles should have all pieces, books should be in good shape (no torn pages), games and activity boxes should include directions and have all the pieces needed to play.

Storage of materials

Store all materials so that they are easily accessible to parents as they enter and leave the center. Staple articles into a folder so that they will be more durable, write the name of the article on the folder, and arrange materials in labeled boxes or on a shelf. If your collection is large, you can organize and label according to the topic, such as Discipline, Nutrition, and so on.

Check-out system

Attach to each item a library pocket or envelope. In it, place a card listing what the item is, with spaces for borrowers to sign name, date, and telephone number. Always have a pencil in the resource center.

Provide a box where borrowers can leave the check-out card. Upon return of the item, the borrower finds the correct card, crosses his/her name off, replaces it in the pocket, and returns the material to its proper place.

If necessary, parents or staff might take turns straightening up the resource center or reminding borrowers to return items.

Encouraging parents to use the resource center

You should be familiar with all materials in the resource center so that you can advise parents to look at the resources that really meet their needs.

Encouraging parents to add items to the resource center will remind them to use it. Whenever parents read articles they enjoy at home, have them clip and send the article in to share with others.

Remind parents about the resource center. Send home a newsletter telling parents about the resource center and how it works. Talk about the resource center during parent meetings. Advertise the resource center with a poster in the classrooms or hall.

Maintaining the resource center

Make sure the resource center, wherever it is, doesn't lose its identity by becoming a catch-all for children's paintings, lost clothing, and extra notices to be sent home. Don't borrow the check-out pencil and forget to put it back. And if the center isn't being used, try to figure out why and redesign, relocate, or update materials. Find out what parents are interested in and be sure to include plenty of materials on those topics.

Make sure you give accurate nutrition information to parents

Parents get lots of information about what their families should be eating. These messages about food come from many sources. Information is often confusing and contradictory.

Many parents are pressured to provide foods that are not the best choice for a family's health. For example, children are convinced that they want to eat sugary cereals or fatty hamburgers because TV advertisements and sales gimmicks are very attractive. Parents may also be influenced about foods from diet plans that are really meant for adults. They may be tempted to feed their children foods that are designed for adults who have weight or health problems.

The nutrition information you give parents needs to reduce confusion so that parents can make good food choices for their families. Here are some tips to ensure that the advice you give is reliable, accurate, and up-to-date:

- Be sure any handouts come from a recognized source, such as the Cooperative Extension Service, USDA, or the American Dietetic Association.

- Look over any nutrition resources to make sure the information contained in the handout is suitable for use by families with young children. If you are not sure, call your local Cooperative Extension Service.

■ Be aware that all resources about food are not necessarily good handouts about nutrition. Check to be sure that nutrition education, not the sale of foods, is really the purpose of the handout.

Respect and enjoy foods from many different cultures

Listen to children when they talk about foods they have eaten that are unfamiliar to you or that you have not tried. Many families maintain cultural connections through diet and food preparation that may seem unusual or exotic to others. Take care to give children a positive message about the foods eaten and enjoyed by their families and let them know that you are always interested in things they enjoy and that you are open to trying new things.

Here are some fun ways to bring foods of different cultures into your program:

■ When you plan cooking projects in the classroom, try to include new foods from families' different cultures.

■ If there are parents who like to cook, encourage them to prepare their favorite foods for the children to try as a special activity.

■ Familiarize yourself with the foods that different religions or cultures use to celebrate holidays. Encourage the parents of the children in your group to share their favorite food traditions or recipes.

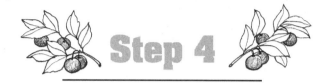

Step 4

Be a Model of Healthful Eating for the Children

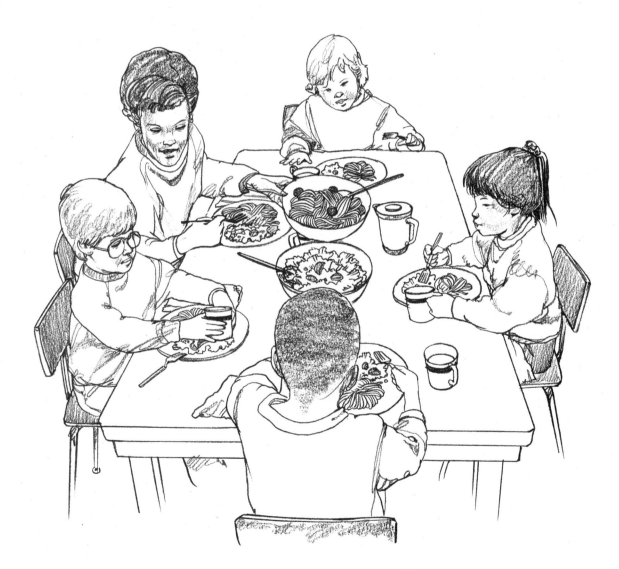

Preschoolers are learning every minute

Preschoolers are learning every minute they are awake. They are learning from everything they see you do or say, from their relationships with others, and from the things they experience in their play and daily routines. Depending on their experiences, they might learn to be curious and excited about learning new things or they might turn off to learning and never want to try new things. Depending on how you act toward them and other people, they can learn to be kind and good at working things out with friends, or they may be unable to get along well with others. The way you handle preschoolers in everything they do while they are with you will have a great effect on the kind of people they become.

Children may not always learn what we try to teach them

Adults often give children confusing messages about what they want children to learn. In many cases, children really learn to do the opposite of what the adult wants. For example, when a child hits another child, some adults try to teach the child not to hit by spanking the child. The powerful message the child gets from this is that hitting is used by adults, so hitting is something that is all right even though the adult says it is not. Children learn their lifelong habits not from what adults say but from what they see adults do and from their own experience.

Children will learn about nutrition from what they see adults doing

Children learn their lifelong eating habits from what they see and what they experience, too. Serving healthful foods will help children learn to enjoy foods that meet their needs for health, but there is more to it than that. Children learn from what they see adults do. Even when adults give children healthful foods to eat, they may see the adults drinking soft drinks or eating other, less healthful foods. Then the children get the message that the foods the adults are eating are really better.

It is important to remember this as you plan to meet children's nutrition needs. Be sure that the children see good examples of healthful eating by the adults who care for them. Then your next step is to provide nutrition activities for preschoolers that will truly be meaningful to them. This requires that you use methods of teaching that work well with three-, four-, and five-year-olds. You must understand how preschoolers learn before you can do a good job of teaching them.

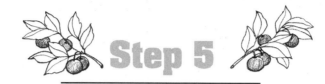

Step 5

Make Nutrition Activities Part of the Daily Learning Environment

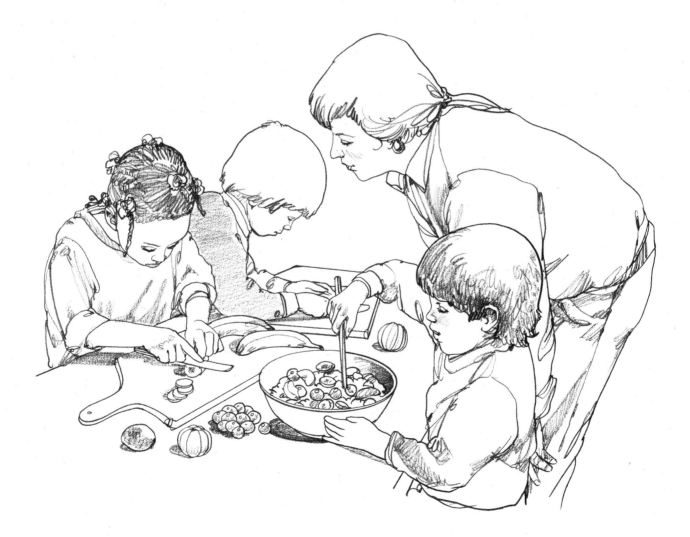

Good nutrition can be taught in the classroom every day

Nutrition can be taught in the preschool classroom most effectively when nutrition activities are part of the ongoing program that meets the learning needs of the children. Instead of making nutrition activities a special one-time thing, nutrition learning can fit into the classroom every day in many ways.

Taking part in the preparation and eating of healthful foods may be the best nutrition lesson a child will ever get. However, there are many other nutrition activities that can be done during play times, too. These activities can have a lasting effect on the good food choices children will make throughout their lives.

First set up a great learning environment, then add nutrition activities

Before adding nutrition activities to a preschool program, you need to be sure that your preschool environment really encourages young children to learn. It takes a lot of understanding about how preschoolers learn to set up this kind of environment. But if the preschool environment is not a good one for learning, the nutrition activities may not work well.

Preschool learning environments must differ from those for older children

The preschool learning environment has to be different from the learning environments of school-aged children or adults. The teachers in good programs for preschoolers realize this and set up their programs to help children learn, using the interests and abilities that the children have at the time. They are careful to avoid pushing children before they are ready. They have realistic expectations of what threes, fours, and fives can do best and build on these abilities.

When working with preschoolers, it helps to remember the following points:

- Three-, four-, and five-year-olds do not have enough understanding of words to make teachers' talking and reading the best way to get information. So, preschoolers should not be taught with long lectures and explanations.

- Preschoolers are just starting to learn how to share, cooperate, and solve difficulties with others by using words to work things out. Good teachers set up areas used by the children so that children can play peacefully, without having to fight over toys and space. They also watch carefully, allowing children to work out the easy problems and stepping in to help with the more difficult ones.

- Preschoolers are working hard to learn to control their muscles, so they do best in environments where they can be active and move around much of the time.

- Preschoolers' learning follows a pattern, and usually one skill in an area of development must be attained before another can be reached. For example, children begin to understand their world based on exactly what their senses (sight, hearing, touch, taste, and smell) tell them. That is why good preschool teachers provide lots of activities in which children can use their senses to learn about real things. They know that school skills like reading, writing, and arithmetic will be learned much better when the child is older and has developed more complex thinking skills.

- To be secure enough to learn, preschoolers must feel safe. Good teachers help children learn to keep themselves safe but realize that young children are not always able to make sensible decisions. They are always present, supervising with interest, and never leave children on their own.

- Good teachers realize that children who feel loved and valued are the children who learn best. They accept individual personalities, avoid comparing children, do not show favoritism, and appreciate each child for all the things that child can do. They help children understand that everyone is different in one way or another and enjoy, rather than discourage, differences.

Encourage free play and active involvement

Since preschoolers are naturally active and curious, they do best in classrooms where much of the day is spent in free play with a wide variety of activities, both indoors and out. Children are expected to be active rather than sit quietly and listen because preschoolers do not yet have the ability to learn well through listening. There are choices for many different activities because the teacher knows that each child's abilities and interests will differ.

Activities should match children's abilities and interests

Activities in well-planned programs are developmentally appropriate, which means that they are challenging but not frustrating, and that there is something of interest for each child. All children in a well-planned program, including children with disabilities, will find many choices for challenging and satisfying activities.

In planning activities, good teachers think about the abilities the children have and then set up interesting activities that match those abilities. They are careful to avoid activities that the children are unable to do because they do not want children to become frustrated and unwilling to try new things. When open-ended materials are used, children are more likely to have success because the materials do not require one right answer. Most of the creative activities in the children's environment should be open-ended.

Open-ended materials are flexible enough that children with disabilities can enjoy and learn from using them just as typically developing children do. This is important because children with disabilities should have play experiences with age-appropriate materials that are the same as those their peers use. Preschoolers with disabilities should not be expected to play with baby toys. Instead, like all

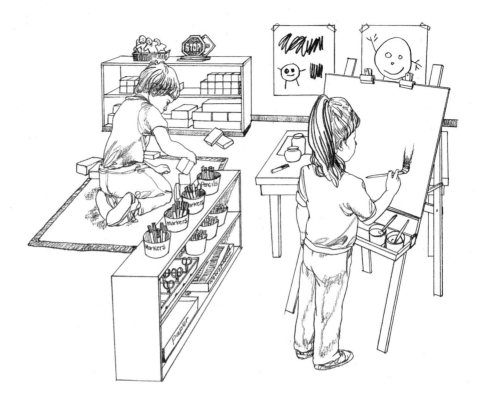

other preschool-aged children, they should be given opportunities to play with preschoolers' open-ended toys and materials in their own way and according to what they are able to do.

However, every good preschool program will have some valuable activities that children enjoy that are not open-ended. Puzzles and lotto or other picture-matching games are good examples of this type of play activity. Many self-help activities, from buttoning a shirt to playing a tape recorder, must also be done in a certain way to get results. Cooking activities must usually be done in one way to get a successful result.

Have many types of activity choices for children

Preschoolers are learning many different types of skills that they will use throughout their lives. They must learn to listen and talk with understanding, think logically, control their muscles, get along with others, do things for themselves. They must also collect an enormous amount of information. Activities for children in an early childhood program should give them a chance to do all this learning. That means that there must be many types of activities going on all day if children are to make good progress.

Organize activities into learning centers

To keep all these activities organized, materials for different types of play and learning can be arranged in learning centers or interest areas. Each learning center is set up for a different type of activity, such as art, books and quiet language games, blocks, pretend play, games with small pieces (puzzles, beads to string), science, and music. The space, materials, and storage needed for each activity are provided. In a good program, the centers are arranged so that quiet activities are not bothered by noisier ones, and many types of play can continue without interruption.

Learning centers require basic materials

A learning center has everything the children need for a certain type of play, including handy storage for the materials, a good space to play, and materials that are neat and organized. The centers are set up so that children can be as independent as possible once they have been introduced to the materials or taught the steps. Tips on setting up learning centers are suggested on page 42.

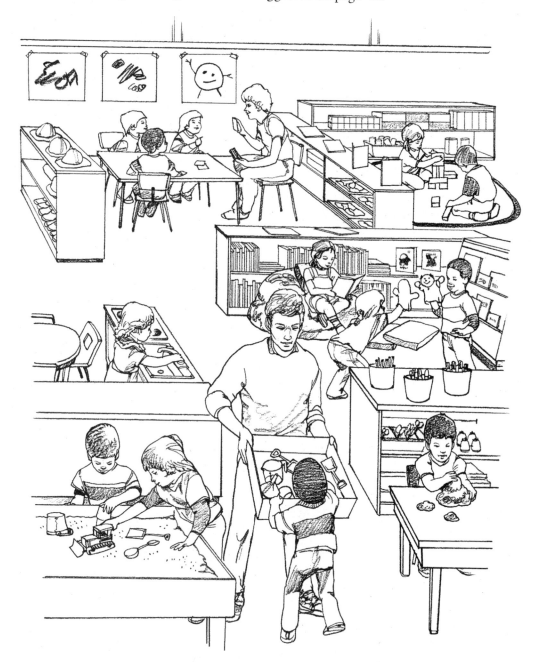

Tips on Setting Up Learning Centers

- Store each game or set of toys in an individual container. Place the containers on open shelves where all children, including those with disabilities, can easily reach them.

- Label the containers with a picture that tells where things go at clean-up time.

- When a new toy or material is put into a center, point it out to the children and show how to care for it properly.

- Have plenty of space for play in each center. Be sure the space is large enough for the number of children who will be using the center at one time. Arrange the play space so that everyone, including those with disabilities, can play comfortably.

- Be sure to have centers for messier play, like art, in an area where water is nearby and the floor can easily be cleaned.

- Set up centers so teachers can easily see what is going on, but clearly separate areas so children can tell one area from another without confusion.

- Make sure that areas are separated so that play from one center does not get mixed up with play from another.

- Arrange spaces so that pathways in the room do not interfere with play in centers and so that children can move about easily while playing. Make sure that pathways accommodate the needs of all children and adults in the group.

- Provide the appropriate furniture needed for play in each center. For example, have tables in the art center or other areas where children need a smooth, hard surface to work on and provide comfortable floor space for activities such as blocks. Make sure that children with disabilities can use the furnishings with their friends.

- Have enough materials in the centers to keep the children busy and interested. Avoid having too few materials or too many in any area.

- Remove toys that children no longer enjoy. Replace them with toys the children have not used in a while or with new activities.

- Repeat popular activities often.

- Have more than one of the favorite toys, books, or other materials so that more than one person can use them at a time. This cuts down on competition and fights.

- Have some activities that children enjoy doing alone and some that encourage play with friends.

- Keep learning centers stocked with basic materials that the children will use and enjoy every day. Other materials or toys can be added to give new life to the center.

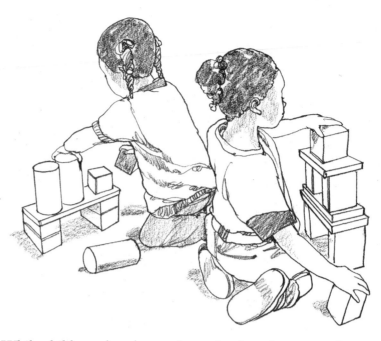

Good teachers use the children's play as a bridge to learning

While children play, the good preschool teacher moves from area to area and helps children or talks to them about their play. She is alert and stops problems before they get out of hand. She teaches by using new words with children, encouraging children to talk, helping children figure things out for themselves, and by guiding them as they gradually work things out with their friends. She notices children's changing interests and growing abilities and introduces new activities based on what she sees. She is always alert to protect the children's health and safety. She watches carefully to be sure equipment is safe, thinks ahead to prevent accidents, and stays close to children who are involved in activities that involve more risk.

The teacher also plans a schedule that meets the children's needs for routines (meals/snacks, toileting, rest time) as well as play. A regular schedule that children can depend on helps children feel secure.

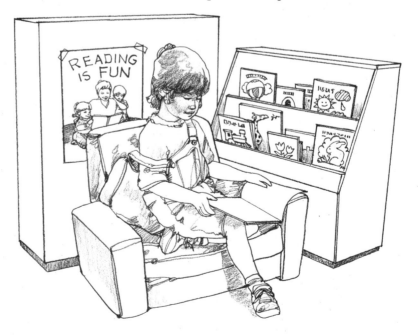

Schedules should be regular yet flexible

Each program will need to plan a schedule that works best for the group of children involved at the time. A basic schedule, such as the one shown, may need to be changed, depending on the season. For example, in the summer, outdoor times might be restricted to early mornings and late afternoons in very hot areas, while some programs may be able to have both indoor and outdoor activities go on all day. Other programs, such as those that serve hospital staff, may need to adjust the schedule to provide the play and routine care activities required for children who are in evening or nighttime care.

The schedule needs to be regular yet flexible enough to provide for a change of pace. For example, the teacher may decide to cut short a group time that isn't going well or move snack time up when children complain that they are hungry.

Sample schedule

Children arrive:	Greet each child and parent Self-directed activities in activity centers
Midmorning:	Wash hands Breakfast or snack Planned play time: self-directed activities for some children, teacher-directed activities for others
Late morning:	Planned large-muscle play outdoors or indoors Gathering or group time: stories, music Routines before lunch (toileting, washing hands) Lunch Clean up after lunch Get ready for nap or quiet time for older preschoolers
Early afternoon:	Nap or quiet play time for children who do not nap
Mid-afternoon:	Napping children get up Routines (toileting, dressing, putting cots away) Snack Planned play time: self-directed activities for some, teacher-directed activities for others Outdoor play time
Late afternoon:	Self-directed activities in activity centers Routines (toileting, getting children's things ready to send home) Talk to parents as children leave
After most children are gone:	Clean up room Set up for next day

Include nutrition activities in the everyday preschool program

A nutrition activity can be added to almost any learning center, as long as it is interesting and enjoyable to the children. You know that children learn best through active play experiences. You can give them nutrition facts as they play if you are careful not to interrupt what they are doing. The information they get as they do interesting activities will be learned in a meaningful way. The following tips will help you teach nutrition facts throughout each day:

Teach nutrition facts through real experiences, conversations, and play

- Have many real experiences with healthful foods, including meals and snacks, cooking activities, tasting activities.

- Talk with children as they eat, prepare foods, or play. Mention nutrition facts during the conversations. For example, if a child sees a picture of milk, mention that the calcium in milk helps us have strong bones and teeth.

- Mention one small nutrition fact whenever it will fit into a normal conversation with children, and you will soon hear the children saying the things you have said.

- Avoid quizzing children about nutrition facts that you are trying to teach.

- Once children seem to know the nutrition fact, move on to another piece of information. Do not ask children to tell you things that they already know too well. For example, when drinking milk, do not ask where the milk came from if the children already know that it came from a cow. Talk about something else instead.

- Be careful not to bore the children with long explanations. Just give a little information and let them guide the conversation.

The activities in the next section can be used to incorporate nutrition into the everyday routine of your preschool programs.

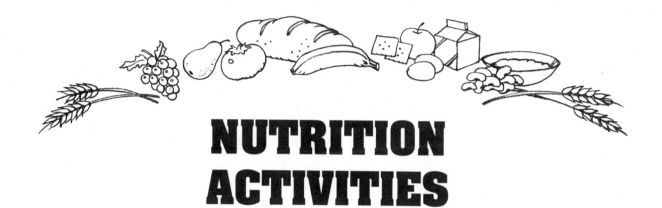

NUTRITION ACTIVITIES

Nutrition Activities
for
Meal and Snack Time

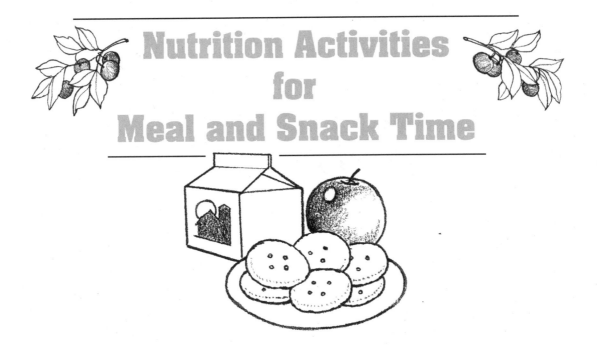

Table Centerpieces

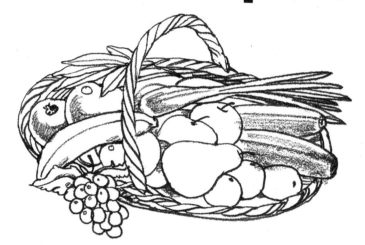

A table centerpiece can add to conversations during meals or snacks. It can be made from just about anything that will fit onto the table without disrupting the meal. For example, seashells, a plant, a play-dough sculpture, or a very small block building might work.

Let children take turns making table center-pieces for the mealtime table. You can help children understand what a centerpiece is by placing one on the table and talking about it at the mealtime.

Our table has a centerpiece on it today. It's in the middle of the table. What is today's center-piece?

That's right, Avie. It's some pretty fall leaves.

Let the children know that everyone can have a turn deciding on a centerpiece for the table. One will be needed for each table every day. Use a sign-up list so that any interested child will be sure to get a turn.

If necessary, put a basket or a placemat on the table to help the child limit the size of the centerpiece they choose. Help the children talk about the centerpieces each day.

Tell us about the centerpiece you put on the table today, Diana. How did you make it?

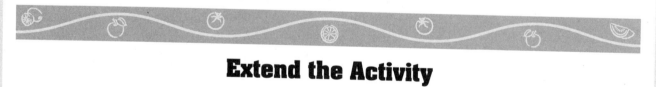

Extend the Activity

- Allow a child to work with a friend to create the centerpiece.

- Make a centerpiece surprise by covering the centerpiece the child has made with a napkin or cloth. Then see if the children can guess what it is.

- Have a week when children choose one special type of centerpiece. For example, there could be a week of centerpieces made of leaves, a week of red things, a week of drawings, and so on.

Mealtime Art Gallery

Help the children set up a children's art gallery near the tables used for meals and snacks. Display the artwork that children have done in this space. Then the children will be able to talk about the things they see there while they eat.

You can use a wall, the back of shelves, a bulletin board, or any other place where children's artwork can easily be seen while children are eating.

Allow each child to choose whether he or she wants to display something in the art gallery. Then let children choose what they want to display. Some children may not want to put up anything, and this feeling should be

respected. Be sure to put each child's name on everything that is displayed, but be sure to ask the child where the name should go.

Change things in the gallery often and talk about the creations with the children during meals and snacks.

I see something new in the art gallery.

That's right, Brian, you made it. Can you tell us about your painting?

Be sure to plan enough time for relaxed meals and snacks so that children can eat and talk without feeling rushed.

Extend the Activity

- Have a guessing game about who did which artwork. Ask children to give reasons for their guesses.

- Ask which pieces of artwork are most alike and which are most different and why. Encourage children to notice details as they make comparisons.

Table Washing

Allow one or two children to help wash the tables before and after meals/snacks. Provide a bucket with a little water in it and a sponge. A towel under the bucket helps catch spills.

Show children how to wring out the sponge into the bucket so that the sponge is not too wet. Then allow them to wipe the table. If the table is especially messy, show children how to wipe the table so that scraps of food, bits of paper, and so on are caught and thrown away rather than knocked onto the floor.

After the children's cleanup, be sure that you always sanitize the table with a bleach solution before it is used for eating.

Extend the Activity

- Let children choose to be either table washers or table dryers. Have wet sponges for the washers and dry sponges or paper towels for the dryers. Encourage the washers and dryers to work as a team to make the table clean.

- Set up a table-washing activity at a small table during play times. Encourage children to practice washing and drying the table as often as they wish.

- Have a damp sponge and paper towels in the pretend play center. See if children wash the table before pretending to eat or feed their dolls.

Practicing Handwashing

Set up an activity so that children can practice the steps of thorough handwashing. Show children pictures of the handwashing steps. You might use the pictures of handwashing steps in Appendix F (page 198). Just copy each step onto a separate card. You can cover the cards with clear contact paper or laminate them if you wish.

Talk about the steps for handwashing, including wetting hands, using soap, rubbing hands together, cleaning under fingernails, rinsing, turning off the faucet with a paper towel, drying hands, and throwing away the towel.

What do you do after you put soap on your hands, Thelma?

That's right, you rub them together.

Yes, it makes bubbles.

Allow interested children to practice handwashing together at the sink. Be sure the children can reach the sink, soap, and towels easily, and that the children are not crowded.

Extend the Activity

- Hang the picture steps for handwashing in the sink area. Talk about them at regular hand-washing time.

- Put up a handwashing picture to remind children to go wash their hands when needed. For example, put a sign on the door so that children can see it when coming in from outdoor play before snack or lunch; put a sign where children will see it after completing messy artwork; put a sign in the cooking area to remind children to wash hands before cooking.

- Place in the games center the pictures that show the handwashing steps. Mix them up and see if the children can put them into the proper order.

Picture Menus

Make food picture cards that can be used to make picture menus for the children to look at. Collect pictures that show the foods children eat for meals and snacks in your program. You might find the pictures you need on food containers, in food advertisements, or in seed catalogs. Ask parents to help you collect lots of pictures, too. Glue each picture onto its own card or a sheet of paper. Label the food with its name. Cover with clear contact paper or laminate if you wish.

Find a special menu place where you can display the food picture cards that show what the children will be eating each day. Have separate spaces for the foods that will be served at each meal and snack. You can divide the menu space into meal and snack sections with different colored construction paper, colored yarn, or colored tape.

Be sure the menu place is down low where children can easily see to talk about the food pictures. Let the children know that they can find out what they will be having for meals and snacks by looking at the special picture menu every day. Encourage them to talk about the foods.

You are finding out what we will be eating today, William. Which foods do you like best?

That is asparagus. We are going to taste asparagus at snack time this afternoon. Have you ever eaten asparagus?

Extend the Activity

- Tell a few children what foods will be served today. Allow them to find the pictures to display for everyone to see.

- Leave one picture off the menu. At meal or snack time, see if the children can identify the missing picture by comparing what they are eating with the pictures they see.

- Put up only the name (not the picture) of one of the foods that will be served. See if the children can guess what the word is while eating the meal or snack.

For example, when carrots, crackers, and milk are served for a snack, you might display the pictures of the crackers and milk, but show only the word *carrot*. Show the children the pictures and the word. See if they can figure out what the word is by looking at the foods they have for snack and then comparing them to what they see pictured on the menu. Give big hints to make the game easier.

Enjoying Foods from Many Places

Help children appreciate the many cultures that make up our society by regularly serving a variety of foods that come from different cultural groups. Foods such as the following can be served at meals or snacks or as special tasting activities: tapioca, which is grown in Thailand and comes from the cassava plant; Hopi fry bread made of cornmeal; Mexican quesadillas or frijoles; scones from Great Britain; steamed rice, which is eaten with chopsticks in Asian countries such as China or Japan.

Talk about the foods and the different cultures that add lots of interesting experiences to our lives.

Today we're having a Japanese soup with very long noodles for snack. It's called ramen.

Who eats ramen at home?
Emma does, and so does Yoshiko.

How should we eat the noodles?
Do you think a spoon will work well?

Extend the Activity

■ Our society uses many foods that have come to us from many places around the world. To help children learn about these foods, you will need to find out about the customs of different cultures. One excellent book that will help you is *Cultural Awareness for Children* by Judy Allen, Earldene McNeill, and Velma Schmidt, published by the Addison-Wesley Publishing Company. Request this book from your public library or purchase it by having your local bookstore order it for you. The book has many activities, including food activities, that can be done with preschoolers and provides teachers with accurate facts about many cultures.

■ Introduce foods from other cultures that the children have not tried before by setting up food preparation activities using those foods. You will find lots of ideas for easy-to-prepare foods from many cultures in the cookbooks listed in Appendix G, pages 200–201.

■ Invite parents to help you plan and carry out a tasting activity that includes favorite foods eaten by the families of the children in your group. Encourage the parents to talk about how the foods are prepared, the ingredients that are used, and how or when they are usually eaten. If possible, let the children help prepare the foods, too.

Healthful Food Displays

Place photographs or posters of healthful foods in the area where children eat meals and snacks. Be sure to include a colorful poster of the Food Guide Pyramid. See if children can tell you when they are eating a food that is pictured on the posters. Talk about where the food fits into the food group sections of the Food Guide Pyramid.

Does anyone see a picture of the foods we are eating today?

That's right, Bryanna. You see a bowl of rice on the Food Guide Pyramid poster. It's in the section with breads, cereals, and pasta.

You can request a copy of the Food Guide Pyramid Poster from your local cooperative extension agent or from the USDA (see address in Appendix E, page 190).

Extend the Activity

- See if children can tell you the names of the foods that are shown in the various pictures and posters.

- Have informal conversations about the foods the children see in the pictures. Help children remember when the foods were eaten for meals and snacks. See who eats the foods at home and find out if any of the pictures show children's favorite foods.

Making Snacks for Parents

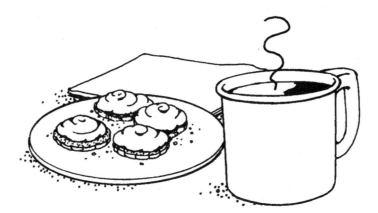

Set up a food preparation activity so that children can make snacks to share with their parents at the end of the day. Be sure to have enough food for both children and adults to enjoy. Some easy-to-make drinks include lemonade in hot weather or hot chocolate in cold weather; simple foods include peanut butter crackers or cinnamon toast.

It's so cold and windy out today. Let's prepare a warm snack to share with parents when they pick you up. What do you think we should make on such a cold day?

Children can decorate the table by using markers or crayons to decorate or by making a special centerpiece for the table. They can even create invitations to invite their parents to the pick-up-time snack.

Extend the Activity

■ Children can prepare familiar recipes for their parents from children's cookbooks listed in Appendix G, pages 200–201.

■ A cooking center can be set up so that children can show their parents how to make a familiar snack by following a recipe from a children's cookbook. The step-by-step single-portion recipes provided in the cookbook *Cook and Learn* are especially good for this type of activity.

■ Children can pretend about cooking and setting the table in the housekeeping area before the parents come to share snacks.

Guess What's for Lunch Game

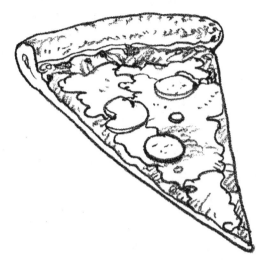

When lunch is cooking or just about ready to eat, have children guess what they will be eating by sniffing the smells of the food. If you use picture menus, be sure to cover them up so that the children will not know what they will be eating. Talk about the foods the children think they are smelling.

Maurice thinks he smells pizza for lunch today, and Elizabeth thinks it will be spaghetti. What do you think, Jonathan?

Extend the Activity

■ Cover one of the serving bowls with paper towels so that children cannot see what's inside. After they have served all the other foods and are eating, see if they can guess the last food that they will be having. Give hints to help the children figure out what is in the bowl.

There's one more thing to eat in this bowl. It's something we eat almost every day. Can you figure out what it is?

It's not milk. You have milk in your cups and you can see it in the pitcher.

That's right. It's bread. This bread is special. It is shaped like a little pocket. Look! It's pita bread!

Recycling to Save Resources

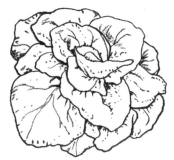 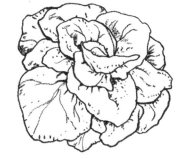 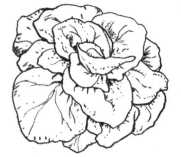

Make it possible for children to take part in much of the recycling that relates to foods in your program. Do recycling activities as a normal everyday part of the children's experience. For example, if your program has a garden, keep a container for recycling fruit and vegetable peelings, seeds, and other unused plant parts for a compost bin. The children can later add these composted materials to the garden to enrich the soil. Talk about how putting foods into the soil makes new plants stronger.

Explain how recycling makes better use of our resources than throwing everything away.

We will not eat these old wilted lettuce leaves in the salad we're making for snack. Who would like to help me take them to our compost bin so that nature can recycle them? The leaves will be turned into food for our growing plants.

Children can also take part in recycling the containers that held foods used in the program, such as plastic milk bottles, glass bottles, and aluminum cans.

Extend the Activity

- Children can recycle some food-related items by using them in artwork that they create. For example, seeds can be saved to use in a seed collage, or cardboard or plastic foam egg containers can be cut up and decorated to string into jewelry.

- Point out when products made from recycled materials, such as paper towels or drawing paper, are used in the program. Help the children remember the things that they recycle as they use these materials.

- Help children understand that paper is made from trees. Recycling paper products means that fewer trees need to be used.

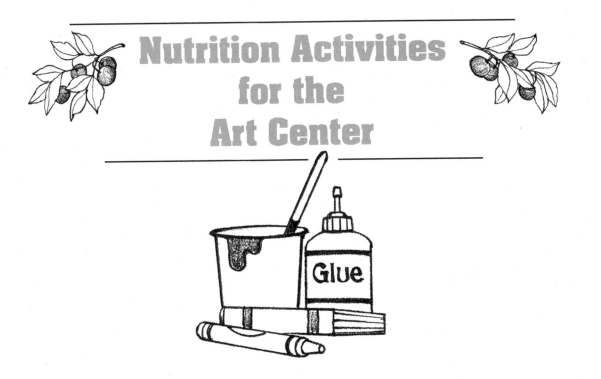

Nutrition Activities for the Art Center

Special Notes on Adding Nutrition to the Art Center

■ **Encouraging each child's creativity is the teacher's goal in a good preschool program.**

Children should be encouraged to think of their own creations rather than instructed to copy something that was thought up by an adult.

In some cases, you may wish to suggest an art project for children to do, such as making play-dough pumpkins to use in the block center or making a favorite foods collage. However, only children who are interested should be encouraged to do the suggested activity, and they should be able to do it in their own way. Children who are not interested should be allowed to use art materials in their own creative way without feeling pressured to do the suggested activity.

■ **Food should never be used as art materials.**

Although activities such as finger painting in chocolate pudding and making macaroni necklaces are popular with some teachers, there are good reasons to avoid these activities.

Children become confused when they are told to eat a food at meal/snack time and then to use it as an art material during play time. This confusion can be avoided when the concepts of food and art materials are kept separate. The real purpose of each should be made clear to young children: food is to eat and art materials are for creating.

The sanitary condition of the food used in art is usually questionable. For example, macaroni or breakfast cereal used to make necklaces is often exposed to plenty of dirt as children wear and eat it. Pudding finger paints are rarely done on sanitized surfaces with hands that have been washed. It's easier to ensure sanitary conditions at meals and snacks or during closely supervised cooking activities than during other play times.

In addition, it is not recommended that food be wasted in creating collages and beanbags; some children may come from needy families that could genuinely use such foods. Wasting food in this way sends a negative message to all children.

Apple Colors Paintings

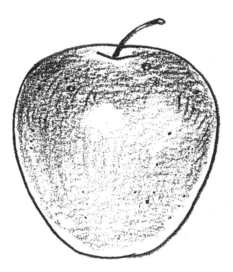

Bring in red, yellow, and green apples for the children to look at and taste. Talk about the different colors, textures, and taste as the children try each type of apple.

You really liked the hard, red apple, didn't you, Sabrina. It was crunchy!

Now what do we think about this yellow apple? Let's try it and see if it tastes the same as the red one.

On the same day, place apple-colored paints in the art area for children to use in their own creative way. Talk about how they are painting with apple colors today.

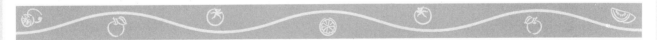

Extend the Activity

■ Allow children to taste other foods that come in different colors. For example, on different days allow children to taste raw yellow summer squash and zucchini squash; red, orange, and yellow tomatoes; red, yellow, and green sweet peppers; brown and yellow pears; pink and yellow grapefruit; or blue blueberries and red raspberries. Provide the colors for children to use as they paint.

Pretzel Art

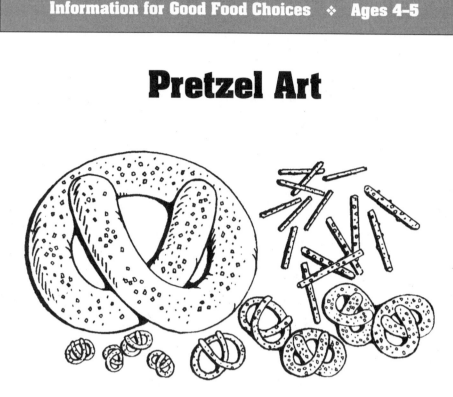

Provide dough for making pretzels, or have each child follow a recipe for a single portion of pretzel dough. (You will find a recipe children can follow to make their own cheese pretzel dough in the recipes section at the end of this book.) Show children how to roll out the dough and then form it into any shape they wish. Each child can place his or her own shapes on a sheet of aluminum foil that is clearly marked with the child's name. Then bake the shapes, which children can enjoy for snack.

Emma, I see you made an "E" out of your pretzel dough. That's your initial.

You made lots of tiny round pretzels, didn't you, Jimmy? Let's count to see how many there are.

Extend the Activity

- Show children different types of pretzels so that they can see the various traditional pretzel shapes. Include large, hard pretzels, twists, large and small pretzel sticks, pretzel chips, and very large soft twisted pretzels. Encourage children to taste all of the different kinds.

- Provide various toppings for pretzels, such as sesame or poppy seeds or raisins. Children can use these to decorate their pretzels in their own creative ways.

- Use bread dough instead of pretzel dough. Allow children to knead and shape the dough. Talk about how the dough changes as it is baked.

Placemat Art

Children can create their own placemats for use every day and also for special occasions. Explain what a placemat is and show some examples to give children the idea. Then provide drawing materials, such as crayons, watercolor markers, or paints, and plain sheets of white or construction paper. Encourage children to create their own placemat designs.

Everyday mats should be covered on both sides with clear contact paper; special mats can be taken home. Children's names should be put on the mats so that there will be no confusion. Some children may be able to write their own names. If they cannot, be sure to ask the child where he wants his name so that you do not spoil the design by putting a name in a wrong place.

Placemats can be stored near the eating area for use at meals and snacks. It's fun to talk about the different placemats while everyone is eating.

Michael made a new placemat today. See the wavy line he made. How did you make that placemat, Michael?

Extend the Activity

- To make special day placemats, provide children with paper shapes to decorate. For example, have pumpkin shapes for Halloween or snowflake shapes for a snowy day. Allow the children to decorate the mats in their own way.

- Show children how to make leaf rubbings for a placemat. Let the child pick out the leaves. Place them on a clear spot on a table. Place paper over the leaves. Then secure the paper to the table with masking tape so that it will not move around. Allow the child to color over the leaf until its shape can be seen. Preschoolers may need to be reminded to press the crayon down hard to get a good print.

- Children can make placemats by placing flat things onto the sticky side of clear contact paper. Be sure to secure the contact paper to a flat surface so that it does not roll up as the child works. Then the contact paper can be covered with a larger sheet of construction paper or another piece of contact paper so that the things are sealed between the layers. Leaves, small flowers, and blades of grass will work well, or small pieces of different fabrics.

- Everyday mats can be decorated with a snapshot from home so that children can locate their places at the table even if they cannot yet read their names.

Making Play Dough Foods

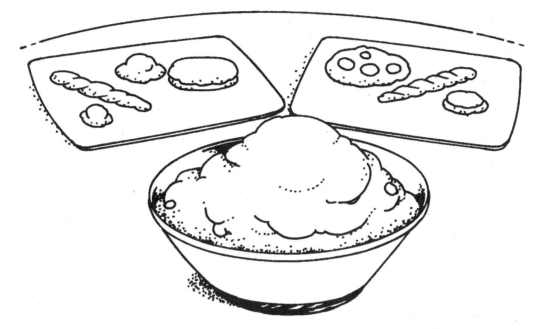

Make play dough with the children. There are two recipes for making play dough in the recipes section in Appendix F. Color the play dough with food coloring to make brown, green, yellow, orange, red; leave some white. Suggest that any children who are interested can make some play-dough foods. Display pictures of healthful foods where children can easily see them while they work. Then let the children create in their own ways.

Some children may want to make play-dough foods as you suggested. Some may create their own fantasy food ideas. Some may want to create other things with their play dough. All of this is great. Talk with the children about whatever they choose to do.

Karen, you are making little round green pieces of play dough. Oh, they're green eggs. They also remind me of green peas.

That's right, Alan. Your brown dinosaur might like to eat those eggs.

Extend the Activity

■ Bake the children's creations in an oven to harden them. See if anyone would like to put a food creation into the pretend play center for everyone to play with. Be sure the children understand that their fragile creations might get broken. Then store the pretend foods in a box on a shelf in the pretend play center.

Making Favorite Foods Collage

Put out lots of pictures of healthful foods for children to glue to a blank sheet of paper to make a collage. You and the children can cut out many pictures from magazines, newspaper advertisements, and seed catalogs. Allow children to choose any of the food pictures to use in their food creations.

Talk with the children about the foods as they work or show you what they have done. See what the children know about how the foods taste and look and when they are usually eaten. Add information about how the foods help us grow strong and healthy.

Tell me about the foods in your collage, Jinsy. Yes, that's a banana. I remember that you like bananas. Are bananas one of your favorite fruits?

Extend the Activity

- Have the children glue the foods onto paper plates to make pretend meals. They can use the decorated plates in the pretend play center if they wish.

- Use pictures of just one type of food. For example, put out fruit pictures so that children can make fruit collages or put out vegetable pictures so that children can make vegetable collages.

- If the child wishes, you can write the name of each food next to its picture in the collage. Have the child tell you the food names to write. Then let the child see the letters as you write them. Spell out loud as you write.

- Some children may be interested in having you write down what they have to say about the collage. Sometimes they may make up stories, and other times they may tell you about ideas the foods give them.

Use a separate sheet of paper to write down whatever the child says. You may wish to use a large sheet of paper for the collage. Fold the sheet in half before the child begins work. The child glues on one side. When it is time to write, unfold the paper and write on the side that is clean.

Do not correct grammar or change the child's words. When the child is finished and you have written everything down, read it back.

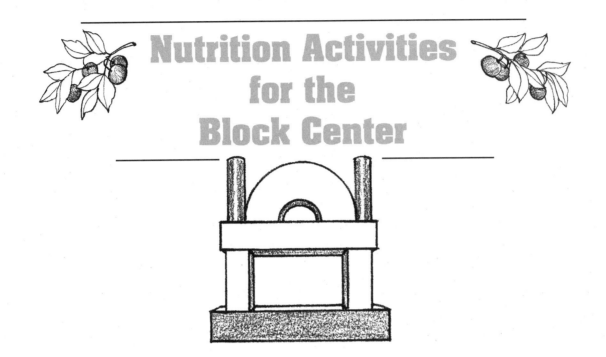

Nutrition Activities for the Block Center

Feeding Toy Animals

As children are building with blocks, see if anyone wants to build homes for the toy animals that are in the center. As they place the animals in the homes they have built, talk about the things the animals eat. Pretend to feed the animals if you wish and see if the children join in the pretend play.

Mention how some of the foods help the animals grow strong and healthy. Ask the children if they eat the same foods the animals eat.

What's the horse eating, Jose?

He's eating grass. Do people eat grass? That's right, we don't.

I bet that horse likes oats. People eat oats, too. Can you think of something we eat that has oats in it?

Extend the Activity

- To help children get ideas about what animals eat, hang pictures in the block center of animals eating. Place them down low where the children can easily see. Talk about the pictures with any child who shows an interest.

- Provide cooking activities in which children use some ingredients that both animals and humans eat, such as oats, corn, barley, and other grains or apples, pears, and other fruits. For example, set up an activity where children make oatmeal or oat bran muffins for morning snack. Talk about how oats are healthful for both horses and people. You can find recipes to cook with children in the cookbooks that are listed in Appendix G.

- When children are eating foods at meals and snacks, talk about the foods that are healthful to both people and animals. For example, when eating carrots see if the children can remember that rabbits, horses, and other animals also enjoy these foods.

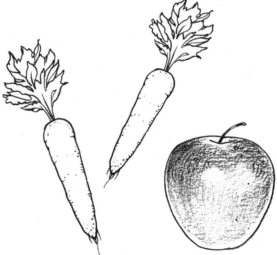

Nutrition Activities for the Block Center

Pretend Foods in the Block Center

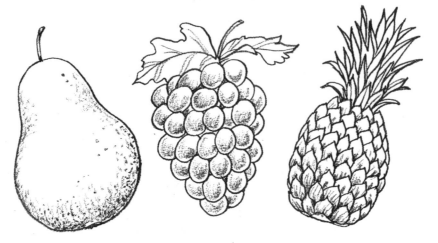

Place a container of pretend fruits or vegetables on the block shelf and see how the children use them in their block play. Provide plastic fruits and vegetables or use foods that the children have made out of play dough in the art center. Watch to see what the children do with the foods as they play.

> *Wow, Amanda! That tomato fills up the whole dump truck! Where is the truck taking the tomato?*

As the children play, talk with them about their play. Talk about what each fruit or vegetable is like. Talk about the fruit and veg-etable colors, whether the foods have skins or seeds, and how they taste. See if the children remember when they last ate the foods. Also take part in the children's pretend play.

> *I bet that pumpkin is really heavy, Brooke. Do you think you need to ask David for help?*

> *Oh! What happened?*
> *Did that pumpkin break on the ground?*
> *There are seeds and pumpkin meat everywhere! How do you think we can get it up so we can throw it away?*

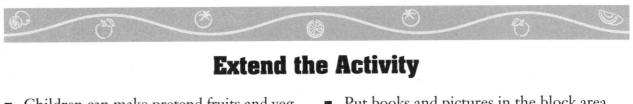

Extend the Activity

■ Children can make pretend fruits and vegetables in the art center using play dough, clay, or papier mâché. Allow children to bring their creations into the block center to use in their play.

■ Put books and pictures in the block area that show fruits and vegetables being sold in supermarkets, being shipped in trucks or on trains, and being prepared in homes or restaurants. Talk about the pictures or read the books with any children who are interested.

Building Roads for Delivering Foods

When you see children building roads and using cars and trucks in their block play, talk with them a little about how people move foods from farms to supermarkets, homes, and schools by traveling on roads. Ask the children if they have seen people delivering food in their neighborhoods. Talk about all the different kinds of deliveries that take place. For example, mention the milk delivery to your program, the pizza delivery car that comes to people's houses, and the huge food delivery trucks that bring food to supermarkets.

Terry, how did you get the pizza you had for supper last night? Did your mom drive her car to get it or did the pizza delivery person come to your house?

Rebecca, your grandmother told me you went to get fresh corn on the cob last night. How did you get to the corn farm?

Pretend to deliver some food to a neighborhood. See if the children will take part by building roads, using cars, and talking about the foods they are moving from place to place.

Extend the Activity

- Ask parents to talk with their children about how food gets to the supermarket. As they pick out different foods, they can tell the child where the food came from before it reached the store.

- Collect pictures of trucks and vans that deliver foods in the community. Hang the pictures down low on a wall or on the back of a bookcase in your block center where children can easily see. As children look at the pictures, talk with them and find out which trucks they can already tell you about. You can tell them about the delivery trucks that are not familiar. Talk about what foods each truck brings to the supermarket. Then listen and watch the children's play with the trucks in the block center to see if their play is about food delivery vehicles.

- Children may want to label their trucks to look like the ones in the pictures. You can

cut out small food store labels or children can draw their own labels for the food delivery trucks. These labels can be taped to the sides of the trucks used in the block area.

- Make arrangements for children to visit a food delivery truck. Try to visit a truck that has a refrigerator to keep foods cold and visit another truck that delivers foods that do not need to be kept cold. Talk about the different types of foods in each truck. Ask the food delivery person to tell the children how the delivery job is done—where the food comes from, the places it is delivered to, how heavy the different foods are, how much food the truck carries.

- Ask parents to help children spot delivery trucks as they drive or walk. Talk about the trucks the children see. See if they can tell what is in each truck.

Grocery Store Block Play

Talk with the children about how cans and boxes are stacked in supermarkets. See if the children can tell you about how things are stacked. Talk about how things have to be balanced so that they will not fall over. See what foods the children can think of that they have seen stacked in supermarkets.

It looks like you're stacking a shelf of cans, Hannah.

What foods are in the cans?

You and any interested older children can work together to set up a pretend supermarket using all kinds of blocks. Ask the children what the different shapes are. For example, they might decide that the big rectangle blocks are cereal boxes and the medium columns are soup cans. You might help children make signs like those they see in the supermarket that tell the customers what foods are stacked in each place. Then the children can sort the blocks and pretend they are supermarket workers stocking the grocery shelves.

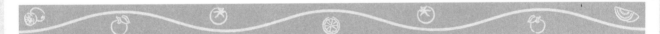

Extend the Activity

■ As children are stocking the pretend grocery shelves, you can talk about all the different foods they are imagining. You can ask questions about what the children do when they go grocery shopping.

■ Use different ways to help children tune in to how things are stacked at the supermarket. You can visit a supermarket with the children so that they can watch to see how things are balanced. You can take photographs while you are shopping and then show the pictures of stacked foods to the children. You can make a stack of boxes in the pretend play center when the children are playing store.

■ Ask parents to send in labels from empty food cans or boxes that they have eaten at home during the past week. Use these labels for the signs that show where the different types of food will be stacked. You may find that some children bring in food labels that other children have never seen or tried. Talk about all the different kinds of foods people like to eat.

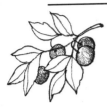

Nutrition Activities
for the
Book Center

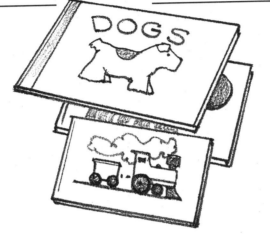

Neat-Eating Book Activity

Read the picture book *Leo the Late Bloomer* by Robert Kraus and Jose Aruego to a small group of children. This book is usually available at your public library and in many bookstores.

When you finish reading, turn to the pages that show Leo being a messy eater. Then talk about messy eating and neat eating. Ask questions such as the following to help children take part in the discussion:

At first Leo was not able to eat neatly. What did he have to learn to eat neatly?

What are some things you can do to eat neatly?

What neat-eating things will you be able to do when you are bigger?

What are neat-eating things that babies cannot do?

Extend the Activity

- Encourage children to act out with movements the different ways messy and neat eaters act. Show children how to do this with actions only—no talking. Have children take turns acting out messy or neat eating while their friends guess which type of eater they are pretending to be. Be ready to laugh at lots of exaggerated antics.

- Help children write stories about when they (or someone they know, such as a brother or sister) were messy or neat eaters. Write down the stories they tell and let them add pictures if they wish.

- At meals and snacks, remind children about how to be neat eaters. Ask questions to help them remember what Leo, the late bloomer, was able to do when he became a neat eater. Avoid pressuring, though, because neat eating skills develop slowly.

Three Bears Table-Setting Game

Read a picture book about Goldilocks and the Three Bears to a few children. Talk about how big each bear is. Then provide flannelboard cutouts of a small, medium, and large table setting, each with a bowl, spoon, napkin, and cup. You can trace the real objects and then cut them out to make the flannelboard cutouts you need. See if the children can make a place setting for each bear that is the right size, arranging the cutouts on the flannelboard.

Which spoon would the mother bear use, Tomika?

That's the one I would choose, too. Which spoon is for the father bear? How do you know?

Some children may prefer not to arrange the cutouts to size. This is fine. Ask a few questions to find out how the child is thinking. You may be surprised.

Why did you give the baby bear the biggest spoon?

Oh! You think he is too small and should eat more.

Store the book with the flannelboard cutouts in a box on a shelf in the book center so that children can play the game whenever they wish. Be sure the children know where the flannelboard is stored.

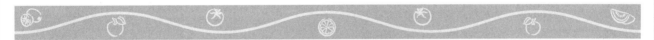

Extend the Activity

- Make big cutouts of the three bears and let children sort the place-setting pieces onto the correct bear.

- Find stuffed toy bears—one big, one medium, and one small. Introduce them to the children as Father Bear, Mother Bear, and Baby Bear. Allow the children to match the place-setting cutouts to each bear, or provide real place settings in the three different sizes for the children to use.

Mealtime Photo Album

Take photographs of children at mealtimes as they do the things that make meals pleasant. Show children being competent and doing things for themselves. For example, photograph children setting the table, serving themselves, using napkins, eating healthful foods, tasting new foods, talking nicely to friends, and clearing their space. Be sure to photograph each child in the group.

Put the photos into an album that has plastic pages so that the photographs will be protected. Place the album on the shelf in the book corner. When children look at the photographs, talk about what each child is doing.

See what the children have to say about the pictures.

That's right, Luis. There you are pouring milk.

What's Catrina doing in this picture?

Can you tell what we had for lunch when we took this photo, Sherry?

Looking at photo albums is often the most popular activity in the book center. It may be a good idea to make duplicate albums by having two sets of prints made when the film is developed.

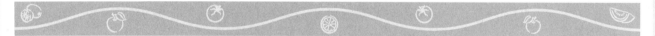

Extend the Activity

- Take photographs of children as they are doing cooking activities. Be sure to photograph the whole cooking sequence. Put these photographs into a cooking photograph album. Then talk with the children about what was cooked, the steps that were taken, and how the cooked foods tasted. Just ask a few questions if you need to get the talking started. Then see how much the children can tell you.

- Ask parents to bring in photographs taken at home during mealtimes. Add these to the photo album. Talk about how home meals are different from those at the program and how they are the same.

- Take photographs of children as they do all sorts of activities. Be sure to include lots of cooking and nutrition activities. Put all the photos into an album. Put the album on a shelf in the book corner and talk with the children as they look at it.

Child-Created Favorite Food Books

Help children make their own books that show pictures of their favorite foods. They can draw pictures of the foods they enjoy or cut pictures from magazines or plant and seed catalogs and glue them to sheets of paper. Cover the books with colored construction paper stapled along the left edge. If you want sturdier books, the covers can be laminated or covered with clear contact paper.

Place the books in the book center. When children look at the food-picture books, sit with them and talk about the foods.

I remember when you drew these strawberries, Lara. It was just after our visit to the strawberry farm. Do you remember what we did with all the strawberries we picked that day?

Extend the Activity

- After the children have created their food pictures, see if they want you to write down what they tell you about the pictures. Allow the children to talk as you write their words on another sheet of paper. Arrange the book pages so that the words are next to the picture in the book and then staple the pages together. Read the books as children look at the pictures.

- Provide cooking activities in which children can prepare some of the favorite foods they put in their books. You will find many recipes that children can prepare in the cookbooks listed in Appendix G.

- Use a loose-leaf binder and punch holes in the paper. Then children can add favorite foods throughout the year.

- Tune into the favorite foods that children showed in their books. When the foods are served at meals or snacks, help children remember whether they included that food in their book.

- Make books of foods of a certain color: foods that are eaten with a spoon, a fork, with fingers; and so on. See if children can think of other food books to add to the book center.

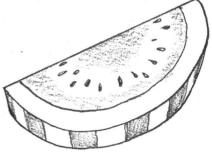

What We Ate for Breakfast Book

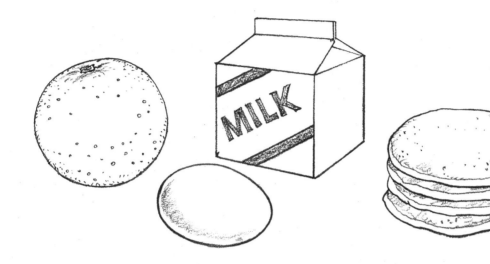

Have any interested children tell you what they ate for breakfast. Write down exactly what each child tells you on a sheet of paper that will be the child's own page in the book. Allow the children to draw pictures or to decorate their own pages in any way they want.

Collect all the pages to make a "What We Ate For Breakfast" book. Cover the book with colored construction paper stapled along the left edge. If you want a sturdier book, the cover can be laminated or covered with clear contact paper.

Place the book in the book center. Read it to children who are interested, talking about how breakfast is needed for energy to play. Name all the different foods that children had for breakfast.

Here's Sandra's breakfast. She had milk and cereal. She decorated her page with lots of swirly colors.

Who did this page? That's right, LaToya. The page shows what you ate for breakfast. It says, "I drank all the orange juice."

Extend the Activity

- You may want parents to help by giving you information about what children ate. Then you can help any children who have forgotten what they ate.

- Make other books about what children ate for meals and snacks.

Nursery Rhymes About Food

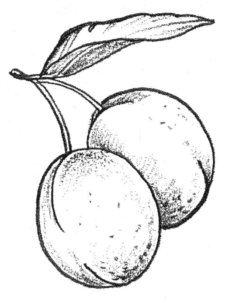

Say or sing nursery rhymes about food with children. Some Mother Goose nursery rhymes about food that preschoolers enjoy include "Simple Simon," "Peter, Peter, Pumpkin Eater," "There Was an Old Woman Who Lived in a Shoe," "Little Miss Muffet," "Little Jack Horner," "This Little Piggie Went to Market," "Old Mother Hubbard," and "Jack Sprat." You will find the words to these rhymes in Appendix I.

These rhymes are often in picture books that you can look at with the children. As you look, talk about the food words and the pictures, too.

Little Jack Horner has a plum on his thumb. We ate fresh plums for snack yesterday. Jack's plum was cooked in a pie. Have you ever eaten cooked plums?

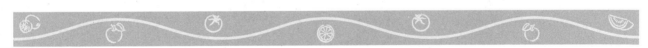

Extend the Activity

- Teach the children to do hand movements with the nursery rhymes. The children may be able to think up their own hand movements, too.

- Clap hands to the rhythm of the nursery rhymes.

- Show children the picture for a rhyme and see if they can say the rhyme without your help.

Cookbooks in the Book Center

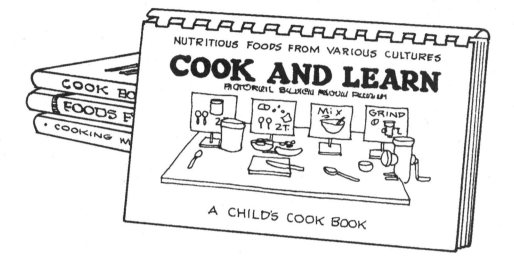

Place some children's cookbooks on the bookshelf in the book center. Be sure that they have clear pictures that children will enjoy. You will find a list of cookbooks for children in Appendix G.

Encourage children to look at these cookbooks whenever they are interested. Talk about the recipes the children look at. Answer questions and read the recipes as requested. See if the children can pick out recipes that they have prepared in cooking activities.

That's right, Antoine! That's the recipe we followed to make fruit salad. Can you remember what the recipe told us to do?

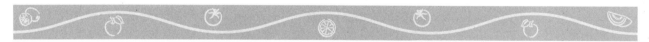

Extend the Activity

- Let the children choose recipes they want to prepare during cooking activities by looking through the children's cookbooks.

- Make a cookbook that has recipes for all of the foods that the children have prepared themselves.

- Include some adult cookbooks that have many colorful pictures. Be sure to include some that show pictures of foods from different cultures.

Blueberries for Sal

Read *Blueberries for Sal* by Robert McCloskey to small group of interested children. As you read about how Sal picks the blueberries, make the hand motions of picking the berries and either dropping them into the pail or into your mouth. Encourage the children to listen closely to the words and to make the hand motions, too.

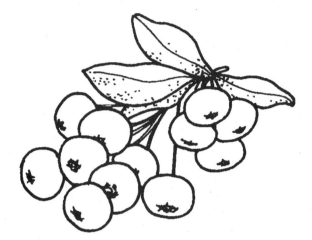

Kuplink, kuplank, kuplunk!

Where did Sal drop the berries this time?

Have blueberries for the children to taste as you read about how Sal and Little Bear eat the blueberries.

Extend the Activity

- Put out a tape of *Blueberries for Sal* with the book so that children can listen and look at the pictures on their own. Older preschoolers will be able to manage the tape player if you show them how. You can purchase the tape and book at your local bookstore, or you can make your own tape, ringing a bell or giving another signal when it is time to turn each page.

- Set up a cooking activity in which children make blueberry muffins or blueberry pancakes after they have heard the story.

- Serve foods containing blueberries at meals or snacks.

- Put small pieces of sponges and blue paint in the art area so that children can make blueberry pictures. They can also use the tip of a paintbrush or a marking pen to make blueberries.

- Children can make play dough blueberries in the art center and let them dry. Then they can put them into blueberry containers from the store or into a bucket like Sal used for the pretend play area.

- Use other children's books about food in the book center. You will find a list of these in Appendix K.

Read and Make Soup Activity

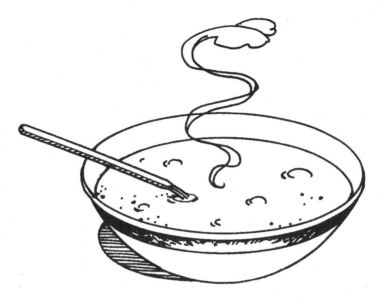

Place the book *Chicken Soup with Rice*, by Maurice Sendak, on a shelf in the book center. You should be able to get the book from your local library or bookstore. Read the book with a small group of interested children. Pay special attention to the poem about chicken soup with rice. Talk about all the different kinds of soups that can be made. Ask children to tell about their favorite soups.

Choose a soup recipe to make with the children. You will find lots of possibilities in the children's cookbooks listed in Appendix G. There are also recipes to try in the recipes section, Appendix F.

This recipe shows us how to make a Chinese chicken noodle soup called "Chi Tong."

Let's look at the recipe to see what we need to prepare the soup for our snack.

Extend the Activity

- Serve chicken soup with rice at a meal or snack after reading the book.

- Ask parents for favorite soup recipes that can be prepared and served in your program. Try to use recipes that come from many cultures.

- Make chicken noodle soup in three ways. Use packaged dry soup, soup from a can, and homemade soup. Have a tasting activity so that children try each one and talk about how they are the same and different.

Reading the Menu

Make a tape for the book center that tells the daily menu for lunch. Put a clearly printed copy of the written menu next to the tape player so that children can look at the words as they hear the menu. Add pictures of the foods on the menu if you wish.

When children have listened to the tape, see if they can tell you what they will be having for lunch. Talk about the different foods.

Did you find out what we are having for lunch today, Daniel?

That's right, fish sticks. You do not like fish sticks?

Maybe you could try them with some lemon or ketchup.

Is there something on the menu that you do like today?

Extend the Activity

- Make a tape of the lunch menus for the whole week. Be sure to clearly state the day for each one. See if the children can figure out which meals they have already eaten and which will be served that day.

- Make a set of food picture cards that show the foods on the lunch menu for the day plus other foods that are not on the menu. Place the cards in a box next to the tape player. Children can listen to the tape and then see if they can find the picture cards that match the menu on the tape.

- Add an item to the day's menu that is not something to eat. For example, record that the lunch for Monday will be chicken, rice, broccoli, a teddy bear, orange slices, and milk. See if the children hear your mistake.

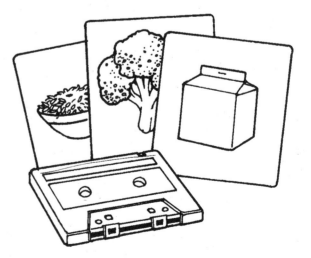

Enjoying Carrots

Read *The Carrot Seed* by Ruth Krauss to a small group of children. This is a great book to read to one or two children. After you have finished reading the book, you can show the children some carrot seeds and a real carrot with its green top. Talk about how tiny the seeds are. Compare the real carrot to the one pictured in the book.

Ask the following questions to help children think and talk about the book:

How do you think the little boy felt when his carrot seed didn't grow?

We can see the top of the carrot. Where do you think the orange part is? Look at the picture that shows the top of the carrot sticking out of the ground before it is harvested.

What do you think the little boy's family thought about the carrot?

What do you think the little boy did with the huge carrot?

Extend the Activity

- Cook carrots and have children try them whole, sliced, and mashed to show children how carrots can change form. The children can help with the cutting and mashing. Allow the children to compare cooked with raw carrots. Talk about how the carrots are the same and different with every change.

- Compare canned, frozen, and raw carrots. Let the children taste them either heated or unheated. See what they say about each kind.

- Plant some carrot seeds in an outdoor garden with the children. Help children notice when the carrots sprout. Thin the carrots and show children the tiny little baby carrots that are growing. The children can wash them and taste them. Pull up a few carrots once in a while to see what progress they are making. Children's interest will come and go over the months that it takes to grow a carrot of any size, but continue the activity with anyone who shows interest.

- Have a crunchy vegetable-tasting activity, using carrots, celery, and other crunchy vegetables. Be sure to cut the vegetables into strips, not chunks or coins, to avoid choking.

Making Stone Soup

Read the book *Stone Soup* by Marcia Brown to a small group of children. Because this is a long book, you may want to tell a shorter version of the story in your own words to younger children.

Children can act out the story by pretending to drop three stones in a big pot, sprinkle in salt and pepper, throw in carrots and cabbages that they have carried in their aprons, and stir the soup as it cooks.

Later, you can set up a real stone soup cooking activity that all children can take part in.

The soup can be served as a meal, snack, or as a snack to be shared with parents at pick-up time. The recipe for stone soup can be found at the end of the *Stone Soup* book and is also in Appendix F.

Provide cutting boards and knives for children to use to cut up vegetables. Make cutting of large, hard vegetables, such as potatoes or carrots easier for children by cutting the vegetables into strips with flat sides. Then let the children cut the vegetables up into smaller pieces and add them to the cooking pot.

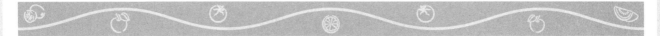

Extend the Activity

- Make picture recipe cards to remind children what goes into the soup.

- Put pretend ingredients for stone soup and a large pot into the pretend play center. Children can then make stone soup for their pretend families.

- Make a flannelboard activity box with all the pieces needed for Stone Soup. Place these in the book center so that the children can act out making their own soup using the flannelboard pieces.

- Place food picture cards that show the vegetables that go into stone soup into the games center, with a big pot. Talk with the children about the foods on the cards as they place them into the pot. You will find the pictures you need to make the food picture cards in Appendix C.

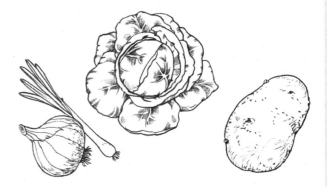

Bread Book Activity

Read the picture book *Bread, Bread, Bread* by Ann Morris to a small group of interested children. As you read, see if any of the children have eaten the breads shown in the pictures. Find out which breads are familiar and which are new to the children. Allow time for children to tell others how the breads taste, where they come from, and how they like to eat them.

You can help by asking a few questions such as the following:

Do you eat the bread hot or cold?

Do you put anything on top? What?

Do you eat it often or just for special holidays?

Extend the Activity

■ Look at the index in the back of *Bread, Bread, Bread* for more information about each picture. You can use the information in the index to give children who are interested more information about the different breads.

■ Make a book about breads to go in the book center. Children can tell you their own stories or thoughts about bread and you can write down their words. Then they can add pictures if they wish. Children might want to tell about their favorite sandwiches, ordering pizza, baking bread at home, or making biscuits from a can. Read the book to any interested children and place it in the book center where children can use it any time they want.

■ Set up cooking activities where children can make biscuits from scratch or from a can, bake bread, or make pizza. There are lots of good bread recipes that children can prepare in the children's cookbooks listed in Appendix G.

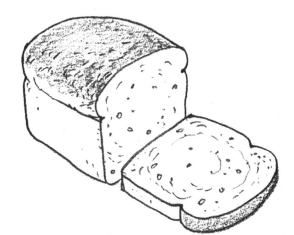

Nutrition Activities for the Book Center

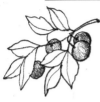

Nutrition Activities
for the
Games Center

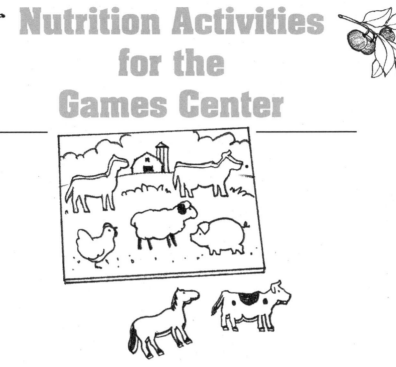

Food Picture Matching Game

Make two identical sets of food picture cards, showing foods from each of the Food Guide Pyramid groups. You will find pictures to copy, color, and cut out in Appendix C. Glue the pictures onto file cards and if you wish, cover them with clear contact paper.

Spread one set of the pictures out on a table or on the floor in a neat row. Give a child the second set of picture cards and ask if he can find pictures that are the same. Have him place each picture next to the one it matches. As he plays the game, talk about all the foods. See if he can tell you the name of each one.

See what else he knows about the food. You can talk about how each food helps our bodies grow strong and healthy.

That's a fruit, Donny. That's right. It's an orange.

Yes! We did have oranges for snack yesterday.

Do you remember how the orange tasted?

Oranges have lots of Vitamin C. They help our gums stay healthy.

Extend the Activity

- Encourage children to sort the food picture cards in different ways. Here are some ideas for how children might sort them:

  what I like and what I do not like

  foods of different colors

  foods that are sweet and not sweet

  foods that are vegetables and not vegetables (older preschoolers)

  food I eat at breakfast, lunch, dinner, and snack

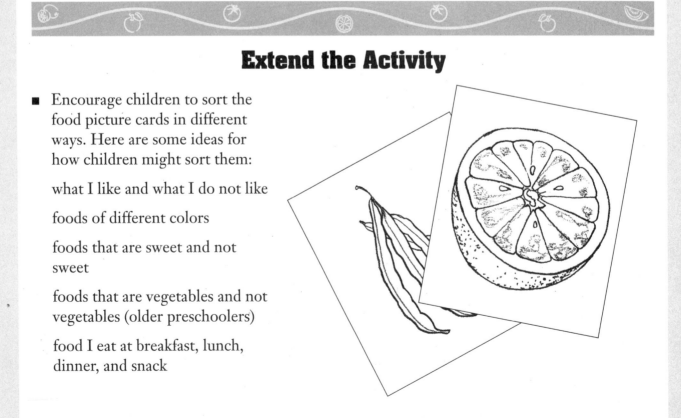

Set the Table Matching Game

Use a permanent magic marker to draw the outline of a place setting (plate, fork, spoon, cup, and napkin) onto a plastic or cloth placemat. If you do not have a placemat, use a piece of cardboard or construction paper and cover it with clear contact paper.

Put the placemat into a box with the real objects you traced. Be sure that all of the place setting pieces are unbreakable. Put the box on a shelf in the games center. Show children that they can place each thing on its matching shape, just as they would do when setting the table. Talk about the objects as the children play the matching game.

You put the cup on its place. What are your favorite things to drink from a cup?

Extend the Activity

■ Make several different placemats with the outlines of place settings that are used in your program for meals and snacks. For example, trace a napkin, bowl, cup, and spoon on one; a plate, cup, fork, knife, and napkin on the next; and just a napkin and cup on the third. Put the three placemats and corresponding objects into the box. See if the children can match the correct things to each placemat.

■ Trace the outlines of small, medium, and large place settings on three different placemats. You might use a doll's place setting with plate, spoon, and cup for the small placemat, a child-sized place setting for the second, and an adult-sized place setting for the third. Put the placemats and their corresponding objects into one box. See if the children can match the correct things to their proper places.

■ Make a placemat for each child with the outlines of plate, cup, and utensils used at meals and snacks. Have all children set their own place at the table, using the placemat as a guide.

■ Gather paper plates, cups, and napkins that come in different sets of matching colors or patterns. Make a placemat for each different set. First trace an outline of a place setting on each mat. Then glue the napkin of each set to each placemat in its proper space. Cover the mat with clear contact paper so that the napkin will not come off. Put the plates and cups into a box with the placemats. Add different colored plastic spoons, knives, and forks. See if the children can match the plates and cups to the napkins with the same color or pattern. They can complete each place setting with knives, forks, and spoons of their choice.

Food Containers Matching Game

Collect two sets of empty cardboard food containers that are familiar to most children. Be sure that the containers held healthful foods and that they are clean and safe. For example, collect two of the same oatmeal boxes, two of the same raisin boxes, two spaghetti boxes, two milk containers, two yogurt containers, and so on.

Take one of each pair and cut out the word or picture that tells what was inside. For example, cut out the big words OATMEAL from one of the oatmeal boxes. You may then throw away the rest of that container.

Place all the uncut containers in a big box. Place all the word or picture parts from the containers you cut up into a smaller box. See if the child can place each word or picture with its matching container. Talk with the child about what was in each container.

That box held spaghetti. I like spaghetti with tomato sauce.

Do you like tomato sauce, too? What else do you like on your spaghetti?

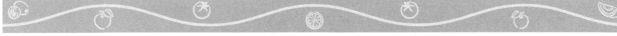

Extend the Activity

■ For children who are just beginning to learn to match, start out with only two or three containers with their matching word or pictures. Help the child figure out how to look for a match by holding up the word or picture next to one container at a time. Ask the child if the two are the same. If the child says "no," then hold the word or picture up to the next container.

Continue until the child finds the container with the matching word or picture. Explain what you are doing as you go through the steps so that the child will begin to understand your system for finding the match. As soon as the child catches on, then let her take over and play the game independently.

Let's see if the OATMEAL word matches this box.

No? O.K. Let's look at the next container. Look for something that looks just like this on this box.

Yes, you found it! This is the oatmeal container.

■ When any of the foods that were in the containers are served for meals or snacks, place the container that held the food in the eating area where it can be easily seen. Have the children guess which food came from that container.

Things We Eat— Things We Do Not Eat

Gather a collection of things we eat and things we do not eat. For example, for "things we eat" include an apple, an orange, a banana, a bagel, a slice of cheese (wrapped in plastic wrap), a cucumber, a tomato, and a green pepper. Be sure foods are healthful and will not spoil if left at room temperature for an hour or more. Since children will be handling the foods, avoid any food that might be messy. For "things we do not eat," include a small doll, a toy car, a small rock, a stick, an acorn, some leaves from a tree, a crayon, a piece of paper.

Put all the things into a bag. Work with one child or a small group. Have children take turns reaching into the bag and pulling out one thing at a time. Then help them sort the things into two piles—things we eat and things that we do not eat.

Talk about what eating really means—putting food into the mouth, chewing, and swallowing. Talk about how the things we eat should help our bodies grow strong and healthy.

Yes. That's a red crayon. Do we eat crayons?

That's true, Sandy. Some babies eat crayons, like your baby brother did. But do big people like you eat crayons? Are crayons a food? Do we eat them?

Extend the Activity

- Make the activity more challenging for older preschoolers by adding things that we do not eat but that are used for eating, like spoons, forks, and plates. When helping the children sort, talk about the difference between foods and things we use to eat foods.

- Use plastic foods that the children play with in the pretend play area as the things that we do not eat. See if the children can sort the foods they really eat from the plastic copies. Talk about which foods should be eaten (or even put into the mouth) and which ones are just for pretending. Use the words *real* and *artificial* when talking about the foods.

How Foods Help Us Matching Game

Make a set of small food picture cards to use with larger "How Foods Help Us" cards. You will find originals to copy, color and cut out in Appendix D. Laminate the cards or cover them with clear contact paper if you wish.

Show children each of the larger cards and talk about how the foods in the pictures help the body grow strong and healthy. Give the smaller pictures to the children and see if they can match each food to its matching picture on the large cards. As they do the activity, talk about the different foods.

That's one of the foods that gives us strong teeth and gums. Where do you think it should go?

That's right! You put it on the picture that shows our teeth. Cheese has calcium and helps our bones and teeth.

Can you tell me about the next picture?

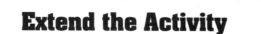

Extend the Activity

■ Make the activity easier by putting out only one large card with its matching food pictures. When the child has mastered matching the small number of pictures, add another large card with more pictures.

■ After children have become very good at matching all the pictures, make the task more challenging by covering the food pictures that are on the larger card. Then see if the children can still remember which foods help the body in each way. When a child has finished sorting the food pictures onto the correct cards, allow her to uncover the pictures on the large card to check for the correct answers.

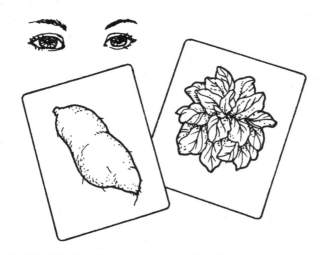

Food Riddle Picture Game

Put out five pictures, each showing a different food. Place the pictures where the child can see and touch them, or let the child hold all the pictures. Give the child clues about each food. See if she can point to the picture you are describing.

This food helps us have strong teeth and bones.
It tastes sour all by itself.
We eat it with fruit.
Sometimes we have it for snack.
It's made of milk.
It's white.

Can you guess what it is?
That's right, Mario. It's yogurt!

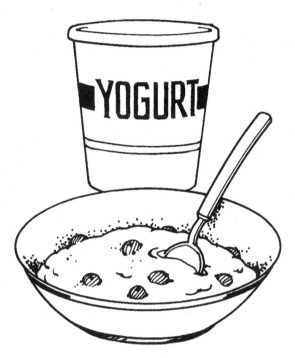

Extend the Activity

■ Increase the number of pictures the child has to choose from as the game becomes easy. Add some new foods that the child is not so familiar with. Or put out fewer pictures for the child who has trouble playing the game.

■ Tape record the clues for a set of food pictures. Show the children how to use the tape recorder. Then let them listen to the clues and choose the pictures all by themselves.

■ See if the child can give the clues while you or other children guess the food that is being described.

■ Have sets of pictures showing the different groups of foods. For example, make a set of vegetable cards; a set of fruit cards; a set of bread, cereal, rice, and pasta cards; a set of meat, poultry, fish, dry beans, eggs, and nuts cards; and a set of milk, yogurt, and cheese cards. Keep each set in a different container, such as an envelope or small box. Let the children choose one or more sets of cards to use to play the riddle game.

Food Picture Puzzles

Make food picture puzzles for the children to use. Glue food pictures to a piece of sturdy cardboard. Then cut the picture into simple puzzle shapes. For younger children cut only a few pieces; for older preschoolers, cut more puzzle pieces. Show the whole picture to the child. Then allow the child to take the puzzle apart and try to put it back together in her own way. Talk about the foods as the child works.

You put two long yellow shapes together, Claire.

What do you think this picture will be?

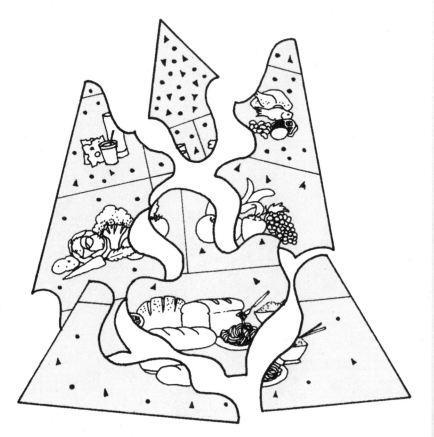

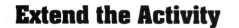

Extend the Activity

- Turn a Food Guide Pyramid Poster into a giant puzzle for the children. Glue it securely to a large sheet of sturdy cardboard. Then cut out each food group section. Talk about the foods pictured in the different groups as the children put the pyramid together.

- For children who find puzzles difficult, make two copies of each picture. Leave one picture intact; cut the other into pieces. Children may refer to the whole picture as they work.

- Make puzzles that show healthful meals.

Seeing Fruits with Your Hands

Prepare several feelie bags or boxes with a different raw fruit in each. For example, put an apple in one, a pear in another, a banana in the next, and grapes in another. Make picture cards of these fruits for the children to look at.

Have the child feel the fruit in the feelie bag and look at the pictures. See if the child can match the picture to the unseen fruit in the feelie bag. Then the child can take the fruit out to check to see if she was right.

Be sure to avoid messy foods in feelie bags or boxes. Talk about the foods as the children guess what they are.

How does it feel, Beth?

It is smooth? Can you tell which picture it matches?

You will find directions for making feelie bags or boxes in Appendix L.

Note: Do not leave feelie containers with foods on the shelves for a long period.

Extend the Activity

- Prepare several feelie bags or boxes with a different cooking or eating utensil inside each one. For example, include a plastic spoon, plastic knife, plastic fork, a pancake turner, a pot holder and a small measuring cup. Be sure all items are safe for children to feel. Provide pictures of the items that are in each bag or box.

  You can put these feelie containers and pictures on a shelf in the games center so that children can play the game on their own.

- Place raw vegetables in the boxes or bags and see if the children can guess what they are feeling. Provide pictures of the vegetables to match, too.

- Have a feelie activity that uses non-messy foods from the bread, cereal, rice, and pasta group. Use uncooked pastas and rice for this activity.

- Put several fruits or vegetables into one large feelie bag or box. See if the children can figure out all the foods that are in the same container.

- Serve foods similar to those used in the feelie experience at meals or snacks on the same day. Talk about the feelie experience as the children eat the foods.

Nutrition Activities for the Games Center

Nutrition Activities for the Music Center

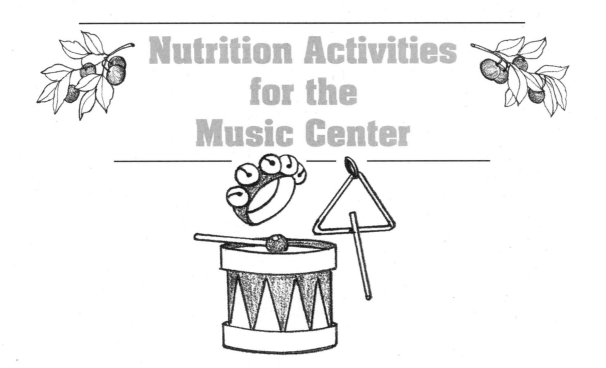

"Old MacDonald" Foods Song

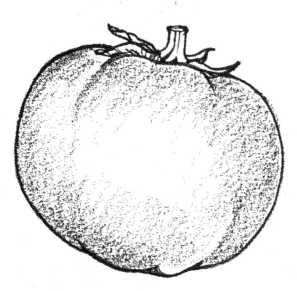

Sing "Old MacDonald" with a small group of interested children, but instead of using the usual words, use healthful foods as the things that Old MacDonald had on his farm. Then use the words "Yum-yum" instead of the usual animal sounds. Give the children plenty of chances to think of the foods they want to sing about.

Old MacDonald had a farm, E-I-E-I-O.

And on his farm he had some tomatoes, E-I-E-I-O.

With a Yum-yum here and a Yum-yum there,

Here a Yum, there a Yum, everywhere a Yum-yum,

Old MacDonald had a farm, E-I-E-I-O.

What food should we do next, Harold?

Extend the Activity

- As children say each "Yum-yum" in the song, add a tummy-rubbing hand movement to show how much everyone likes eating the healthful food.

- Use food picture cards to tell the children the name of the food that you will be singing about. Hold up the food picture at the beginning of each verse and then see if they sing the name of the food.

"Stir the Soup" Songs

Sing a food song that the children help you make up using the tune for "Row, Row, Row Your Boat." Instead of using the usual words, sing these words instead.

Stir, stir, stir the soup

Stir it all day long

Add some _____,
　　　　　　[fill in healthful food name]

Take a taste.

Soup will make us strong.

Let children take turns filling in the names of foods that will go in the soup. Do not worry if the food names they suggest do not make sense. Allow them to say any food they want and everyone can laugh together as the soup becomes a silly soup.

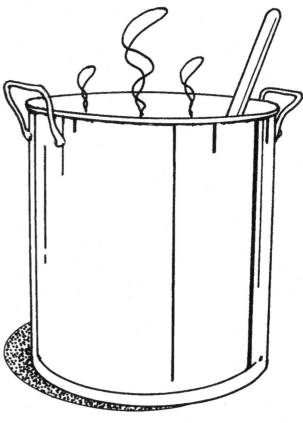

Extend the Activity

- Add movements to the song. Use stirring motions for the first two lines. Then use a throwing motion for line three, a tasting motion for line four, and a motion that shows arm muscles for the last line.

- Use food picture cards to help children identify foods to add to the soup.

- Do a soup-cooking activity in which children can add some of the foods they sang about.

"This is the Way We Eat Our Food" Song

Sing a food song with a small group of interested children using the tune to "This is the Way We Wash Our Clothes." Instead of using the usual words, use words that tell about healthful, familiar foods. Let children tell you the foods they want to use in the song, as well as the name of the meal or snack time when the food would be eaten.

This is the way we eat our cereal,
[pretend to eat]

Eat our cereal, eat our cereal,

This is the way we eat our cereal

At breakfast in the morning.

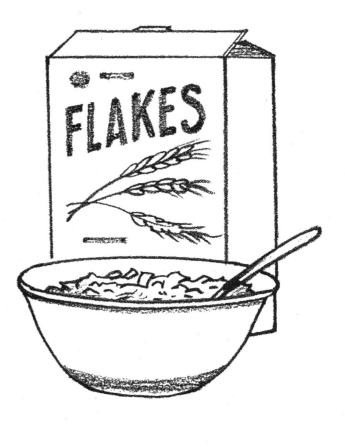

Extend the Activity

■ Include foods that can be eaten with the hands or with a fork, or liquids that we drink from a cup. Help the children figure out how to act out the motions.

■ Pretend to eat very cold or very hot foods and act out how people's faces look when they bite and chew these foods.

■ Exaggerate the motions of eating foods like peanut butter (sticks to the roof of your mouth), spaghetti (is so long you can't fit it in your mouth), or peas (which fall off the fork or spoon).

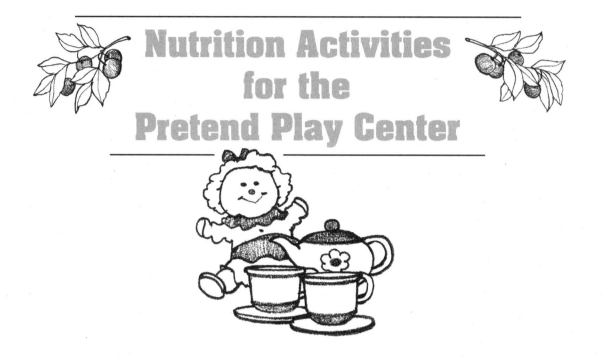

Nutrition Activities for the Pretend Play Center

Special Notes on Nutrition Activities for the Pretend Play Center

- **Have many healthful pretend foods for children to play with.**

  Be sure to have lots of choices in the pretend play foods that children can use. If you choose to include pretend hamburgers, hot dogs, and french fries, be sure that you also make available lots of pretend fruits, vegetables, breads, cereals, milk products, and lean meats.

- **Talk with the children about healthful foods as they play, but avoid turning the play into a lesson or a quiz.**

  Too much structure interrupts play and turns off the children's enjoyment of learning.

- **Be accepting of children's enthusiasm about foods that are considered to be less healthful.**

  Enjoy their pleasure when they talk about fast food restaurant or party experiences, but encourage children to talk about pleasurable experiences with healthful foods often.

Pretending to Prepare Favorite Foods

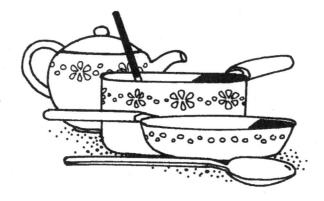

Encourage children to think of their favorite foods and then to pretend to prepare them. You can start this kind of play by acting out food preparation while you talk about what you are doing.

My favorite food is pizza.

I think I'll make some to eat for lunch.

I need to make the dough and the sauce, and grate some cheese.

Talk about the favorite foods as the children play. For example, talk about which ingredients they need, what steps to follow, and what utensils and equipment are needed.

Jeff, do you have enough eggs for your cheese omelet? What else do you need?

Sarah, this lemonade is delicious. How did you make it?

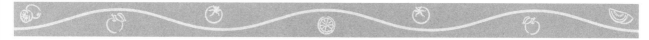

Extend the Activity

- You can read the menu for the day so that children can pretend to prepare the snacks or meal.

- Children can pretend to write their favorite recipes on cards and put them in a recipe box to use in their pretend play kitchen.

- Find used cookbooks that you can add as props for pretend play. The children can then pretend to look up their favorite recipes, or you can really look them up and read what the book has to say.

Setting the Table for Pretend Meals

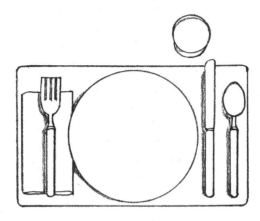

Place sturdy, realistic toy plates, cups, knives, forks and spoons in the pretend play center. These may be neatly stored in a box that has a picture label to show where the things go at clean-up time. Include some placemats onto which place settings have been outlined. Show children how the placemats help them set the table with all the things they will need for their pretend meals.

Are you cooking the supper, Tran?

Let's set the table, Emily, so we will be ready to eat when Tran has our supper ready. Who is going to eat supper with us? How many place-mats do we need?

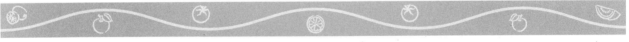

Extend the Activity

■ As you take part in the pretend play, ask children to help you set a place for a meal or snack. Tell the children that you will be having a certain food for your meal, for example, soup or cereal with milk. Then see if they can figure out what things you will need for your place setting in order to to eat those foods. See if they can set places for a cold drink of milk, a plate of spaghetti, an apple that needs cutting, and other favorite healthful foods.

■ Give children a chance to help you set the place for healthful foods they choose to pretend to eat.

Feeding Baby Pretend Play

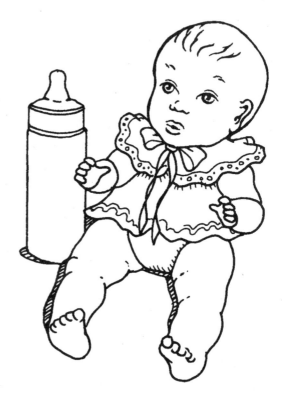

Include lots of things in the pretend play center that are used for baby feeding. Include empty containers from baby foods, such as baby cereal boxes and baby juice cans. Remember to avoid glass containers. Make sure that there are no sharp edges and that the containers are clean. Include real plastic baby bottles and dishes as well as small baby spoons, too.

When the children play with dolls, talk about the foods that are usually fed to babies. Explain how the different foods help babies grow strong and healthy.

You're giving the baby her bottle, aren't you Deirdre?
That's right, the baby likes her formula.

Baby formula is like milk. But it has extra ingredients in it that help baby grow. What else do you feed your baby?

Extend the Activity

■ Talk about the special things that need to be done to feed babies. Have the children try to figure out why bottles are used, as well as small spoons and soft foods. If you wish, you might talk about breast feeding as a very healthful way to feed a baby.

Pretending with Empty Food Containers

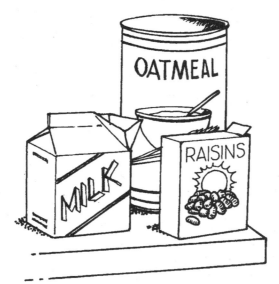

Place empty food containers on a shelf in the Pretend Play Center. Be sure that the containers are those that held healthful foods. For example, include containers that held oatmeal, raisins, milk, and orange juice rather than cake or brownie mixes or salty snack foods. Avoid using glass containers. If you use empty cans, be sure that the edges are not sharp. Make sure that all containers are clean.

Allow the children to use the containers to pretend as they play house. Talk about the foods that were in the containers as you pretend with the children. See what they say as they play.

Yes, Michael, I'd love some breakfast. Yummy! Oatmeal is good. I'm glad you're fixing some oatmeal for our breakfast.

Extend the Activity

- Include plastic or other artificial fruits and vegetables in the pretend play center. As children play, talk about how these taste, look, and grow.

- Make a shopping list to use for pretending to go to the store. Let children think about meals they want to have and then write

down the foods they suggest to buy. Talk about how all the healthful foods they suggest help them grow strong and healthy and taste good, too.

- Read a little bit of the nutritional information found on the boxes to interested

continued on next page

Pretending with Empty Food Containers (continued)

children. For example, look up how much iron is in a serving of Cream of Wheat®. Let them see that you are getting information from the box. Show them where you are reading if they want to look.

Avoid going into details with the children, but tell them a little about what is in the food and how it helps your body grow strong and healthy. In this way you will model how to read to find out how healthful foods really are.

> *Wow! The box says this Cream of Wheat has lots of iron in it. I'm going to eat it for breakfast so that my blood will be really strong. Do you want to help me cook it, Angela?*

■ Provide paper grocery bags that are full of pretend foods and other items that are bought at the supermarket. You can use plastic pretend foods, clean empty food containers, or picture cards that show fresh fruits and vegetables, ice cream in the carton, cereal in boxes, bottles of milk. Encourage the children to pretend to put groceries away.

> *Oh, you got some Cheerios®, Martha. Where do you want to put that cereal?*

> *James, this frozen yogurt is melting. Are you going to put it in the freezer or will you serve us some for snack?*

> *These grapes look delicious, Tyrone. Do you want to wash them before you put them away?*

■ Provide children with clean, safe, empty nonfood containers such as laundry detergent, dishwashing liquid, or pet foods. Talk about the things people eat and things they don't eat as the children play.

■ Set up a little grocery store where children can play. Place this near the everyday pretend play center so that children can go from one to the other easily, without disrupting the play of others. Use a small shelf for empty food containers, a little table with one or more cash registers, and some paper grocery bags or reusable cloth or mesh bags. Add plastic fruits and vegetables as well as other plastic foods that are healthful. Allow the children to make play money if they are interested, or provide some that you made or bought. If there is room, include one or more child-sized shopping carts.

Pretending with Cooking and Eating Utensils from Many Cultures

Add cooking and eating utensils from many cultures to the more typical food preparation and eating materials in the pretend play center. For example, provide various types of chopsticks and bowls, a small wok, rice-serving utensils, a rice steamer, baskets for steaming vegetables and other foods, and teacups from Asian cultures; baked clay dishes and pots, a tortilla press, and baskets for carrying food from Mexico; and bowls and cups made from wood or gourds from African cultures. Encourage the children to use all the different utensils in their own creative ways as they pretend. You can tell and show them how the items are used.

I see you are using the rice steamer, Shelly.

Here's the rice paddle for scooping the rice into the bowls.

As you add each item, be sure you know exactly which culture it is from, what it is called, and how it is used. You will need this information to give children an accurate idea of how people in different cultures do things. Remember that utensils used in one culture may not be used at all in another culture that is located in a nearby area. For example, cooking and eating practices differ from one Asian culture to another.

Extend the Activity

- Ask parents to help you build the collection of cooking and eating utensils for the pretend play center. Have them bring in the utensils and tell any interested children about them or to demonstrate how they are used.

- Provide books that show pictures of people using the utensils or tell stories about cooking from different cultures.

- Do real cooking activities in which the children use the utensils.

- Include clean, empty food containers that held foods used by people of varying cultures. For example, try to provide empty rice bags with Chinese or Japanese printing on them that you can stuff with crumpled newspapers and empty boxes and cans from Mexican, Puerto Rican, Jewish, Italian, or Chinese foods that can be found in specialty areas of many supermarkets. Be sure to ask parents to help you with collecting these props for children to use in their play.

Pretend Play about Foods That Do Not Come From the Supermarket

Put up pictures in the pretend play center of people who are fishing, gardening to grow fruits and vegetables, picking wild berries or nuts, or getting foods in other ways that are different from supermarket shopping. Talk with the children about how these are ways that some people can get foods without going to the supermarket. See what the children can tell you about any of these methods of finding foods. Make sure the children understand that these things must only be done with adults who know what is safe to eat.

Provide props in the pretend play center so that children can act out fishing, gardening, berry picking and other ways to get foods. For example, provide a pretend fishing rod that has a short line with a magnet on the end to catch paper fish that have paper clips attached. Provide a fisherman's basket for the catch. Or provide baskets that the children can carry as they harvest a pretend garden or find wild berries, apples, or nuts. Be sure to have more than one of the most popular props so that children do not have to wait long to get a turn.

It looks like you are all ready to go fishing, Tiffany.

Are you going to fish in the river where your grandmother fishes?

Maybe we can cook the fish you catch for dinner.

Extend the Activity

■ Read books to the children that tell about gathering berries, fishing, and gardening. Ask the librarian at your public library for help in finding easy picture books about these topics.

■ Take a field trip to a farmer's market in your area or see if you can visit a child's home where the family has a garden for growing food. Talk about the differences between getting foods in these places and in a supermarket.

Going on a Pretend Picnic

Have a picnic lunch or picnic snack time with the children in your group. Talk about what having a picnic means. Let the children talk about picnics so that they can share information with one another and you can add new information to what they already know. Display pictures of people having outdoor picnics and put books out for children to look at that tell about fun picnic experiences. Ask your local librarian for help in choosing very easy picture books on this topic.

Once the children seem to understand what picnics are all about, gather together the props that are needed for picnic pretend play. For example, include colorful napkins, plastic forks, knives and spoons, a thermos, a blanket to sit on, and a big picnic basket. See if the children pretend to go on a picnic as they use these things.

Encourage children to work together to plan the foods and drinks they want to take with them and how many will be going on the picnic. Talk about where the children plan to have their pretend picnic.

I see you are putting carrots into the picnic basket, Sachi.

What else will you need?

Extend the Activity

- Let children plan the menu and prepare the food for a real picnic.

- Find out about how picnics are carried out in different cultures—what foods are served and how the foods are packed. Parents may be able to help by giving you information that you need. For example, Japanese people place foods, such as rice rolled in seaweed, in small boxes called *bento*. The bento are then wrapped in scarves to be carried on a picnic.

- Play a record or tape of the old song, "The Teddy Bears' Picnic." Then add toy teddy bears to the picnic props in the pretend play center and see if the children use them in their picnic play.

- Gather the props needed for picnics of many cultures and include them in the pretend play center. You can explain to the children about how the new props are used, or a child who is familiar with the props may be able to tell others about them.

Nutrition Activities for the Pretend Play Center

Nutrition Activities for the Science and Math Center

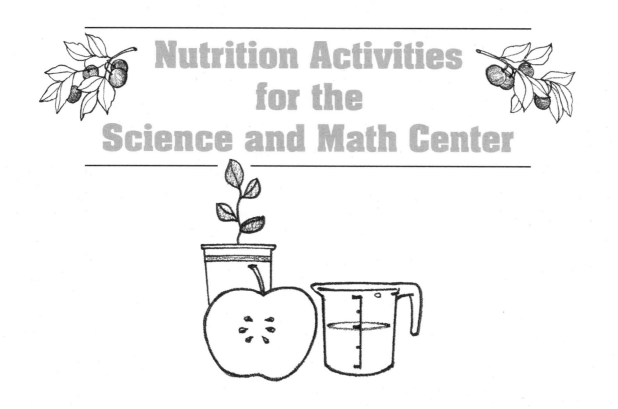

Special Notes on Nutrition Activities for the Science and Math Center

- **Make science activities as hands-on as possible for children.**

  Organize things so that all children can do everything for themselves. For example, when looking at seeds in a banana, allow each child to slice a piece of banana with a knife and then look for the seeds.

- **Do food activities in small, informal groups.**

  Avoid large groups so that children will not have to wait for long periods or have trouble seeing what is going on. If needed, have a waiting list for children to sign up on. You can write their names and then explain that their name will wait while they take part in other fun activities in the room. Repeat the activity until all children on the list have gotten a chance.

- **If foods are to be used in an activity, be sure that all children will be able to taste while they explore.**

  Have sufficient quantities for all who might be interested.

- **When exploring foods in the Science and Math Center, use the same sanitary practices that are used in regular food preparation and serving.**

  Make sure that everyone washes hands before handling foods and that the table is clean. Be sure that foods are cut with clean utensils. Be sure that each child eats only the food that he or she has handled.

- **If activities with tasting are done with children who are three or younger, take special care to avoid foods that may cause choking.**

- **Talk with the children about healthful foods as they come up in their explorations. However, avoid turning the activities into a lesson or a quiz.**

- **Use lots of real cooking activities with children so that they can explore foods in many ways.**

Every cooking activity that children do will also be a science and math activity. Recipes are provided in Appendix F; cookbooks for use with children are listed in Appendix G.

Fun Pouring Practice

Set up water play with real cups and small pitchers. You can add these things to a water table for several children to use or to dishpans that can be used by one child at a time. Be sure that all pouring containers are unbreakable.

Set up the water play in a place where spills can be cleaned up easily. Protect the floor with newspapers, an old shower curtain, or other covering if needed.

Talk with children as they practice pouring while they play. Describe what they are doing. Give them plenty of time to tell you about what they are doing, too.

Wow, Andre! You filled the cup right up to the top. It's really full.

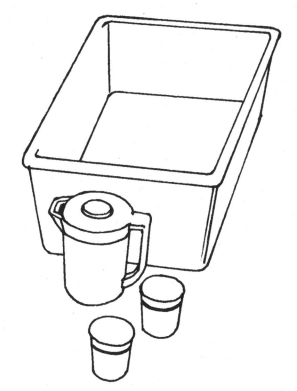

Extend the Activity

- Mark some see-through plastic cups with lines at different levels. Challenge any interested children to get the water as close to the line as they can. Allow children to put their own lines on the cups if they want.

- Have cups and pitchers of different sizes— some large, some medium, and some very small. Allow the children to use these cups and pitchers freely.

- Add safe large containers used for the drinks served to children, such as gallon plastic milk jugs or large pitchers. Allow children to fill and empty these containers.

- Move the water play outdoors on nice days.

Nutrition Activities for the Science and Math Center

Water Play with Sponges

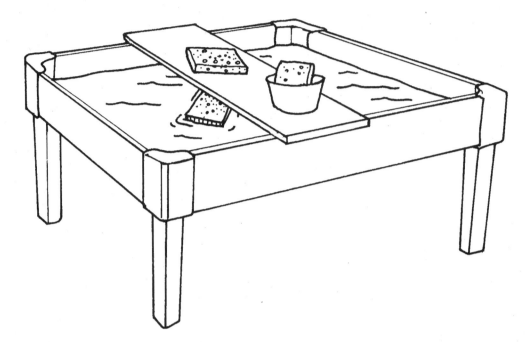

Add some sponges to the water table or dish-pans used for water play. Allow children to experiment with them in their own way.

Talk about how the sponges soak up water and how the water can be wrung out. Show the child how to squeeze the sponge until it is empty. Remind the children that sponges are useful tools for cleaning up spills.

We use sponges to help clean up sometimes. Can you remember when we used a sponge?

That's right. You spilled your juice and used a sponge to wipe it up. And we used another sponge to clean up the paint that spilled.

Extend the Activity

- Have sponges of different sizes for the children to use. Add cups into which the children can squeeze the liquid from each sponge. They can then compare the water in the cups to see which sponge holds the most water.

- Have sponges made of different materials, such as natural sponges and plastic sponges. Allow the children to experiment with the sponges in their own way.

Serving Practice with Sand

Put unbreakable serving spoons and bowls and some unbreakable plates in a sand table or dishpans that contain sand. Allow several children to play with these things at the sand table (or one child at each dishpan). Talk about how the serving utensils are used at meals and snacks. Let the children practice by playing with the things in their own way.

What foods do you like serving with spoons like these?

Yes, you like serving peaches because they are your favorite fruit, Trina. Can you think of a food that is hard to serve with a spoon?

Dishpans can be placed into larger shallow boxes or onto trays to catch some of the sand that is likely to fall. Have a broom and dustpan handy to clean up spills. A child-sized broom or whisk broom will make it possible for children to help with cleanup.

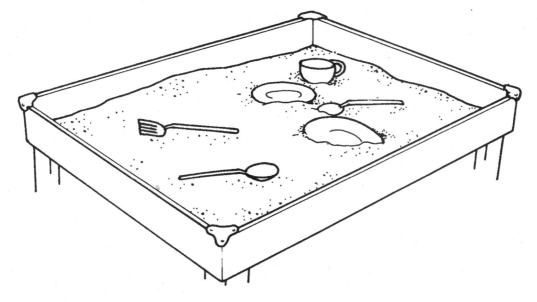

Extend the Activity

- Add some more unusual serving spoons, such as soup ladles or slotted spoons.

- Put plastic foam packing chips into the dishpans or table. Then let the children practice using the serving utensils.

- You might add the serving things to the outdoor sandbox, but collect them at the end of the play period.

Nutrition Activities for the Science and Math Center

Food Group Tasting Activities

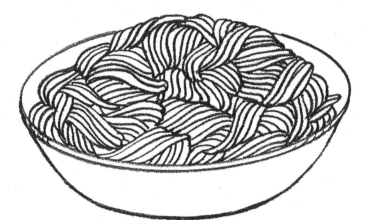

Have a tasting activity in which children have a tiny taste of a variety of foods that come from one of the food groups. For example, have a bread, cereal, rice, and pasta food-tasting activity and provide several samples of each of these foods. As the children taste a little of each food, talk about how they help our bodies, where they come from, and how the foods taste. Be sure to name foods that are not familiar to the children and talk about their taste, color, and texture. Encourage children to tell what they know about the foods.

These foods are all made from grains that grow on farms.

They help our bodies grow strong and healthy.

This pasta is called linguini.

How does it feel when you eat it?

Slippery?

Rhoda says she eats linguini with cheese at her house.

Remember: In a tasting activity, children are given to chance to taste tiny samples of several foods. Be sure that the activity does not fill up children's stomachs so much that they will not eat regular meals or snacks. Children should be offered a sample and encouraged but never forced to try each food.

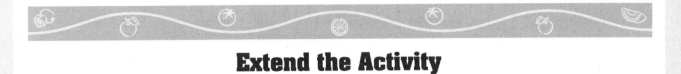

Extend the Activity

■ Have tasting activities in which children taste foods with a specific feature in common. For example, children can sample vegetables that grow under the ground, like carrots, radishes, turnips, and potatoes.

Tasting Foods in Different Forms

Have a tasting activity in which children taste tiny samples of one food that has been prepared in several ways. For example, provide cooked white rice, cooked brown rice, cooked wild rice, rice cakes, puffed rice cereal, and fried rice, and offer the children a small taste of each. Show the children the different types of uncooked rice, too. Or provide an apple tasting activity so that children can taste little samples of apple juice, raw apple slices, apple sauce, and dried apple slices.

Talk about how each form of the food is the same or different from the others.

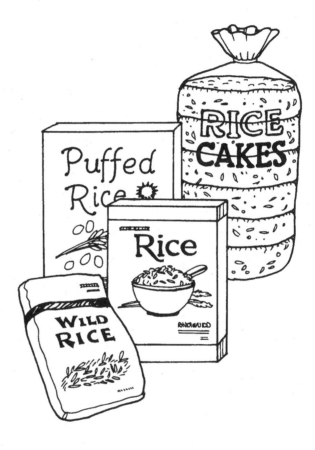

Which rice was crispy?
Which was soft?

The wild rice was chewy, wasn't it?
Which kinds of rice did you like the best?

Extend the Activity

- Set up a series of cooking activities so that the children can prepare the same food in several different ways. These can be done on different days of the week. Allow children to repeat preparing their favorites many times and have them for snack.
- When different forms of food are served for meals or snacks, talk with the children about the other ways the same food has been prepared.

This is fried rice made with vegetables and scrambled eggs that we're having for lunch.

Do you remember other kinds of rice that we eat?

Feeding Birds
(and Squirrels, too!)

Help the children watch any birds that live near your program to see what they eat. The children may see the birds eat berries from trees or bushes, or seeds from a bird feeder. Talk with children about foods that different birds eat. Compare the bird foods to the foods eaten regularly by the children.

Roy saw a robin catch a worm this morning!
Robins eat lots of worms.
Do we eat worms, too?

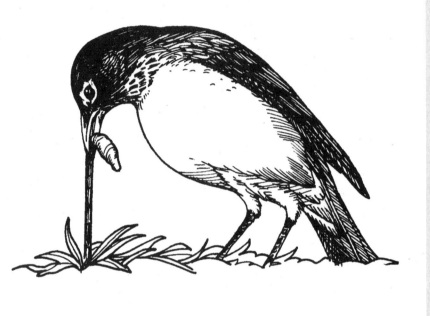

Extend the Activity

■ Plan activities that allow the children to feed birds (and usually any squirrels that are nearby, too!) Children can help prepare foods for the birds. Here are a few bird foods that children can make:

Mix peanut butter with cornmeal, making sure to add enough cornmeal so that the mixture is not too sticky. The children can put the peanut butter/cornmeal mixture on pinecones and hang the pinecones from

branches outside a window where the children can see.

Provide water nearby for the birds to drink.

String popcorn and orange slices to hang outside on branches.

Put dried corn out for the birds.

Fill a bird feeder with sunflower seeds.

Mix leftover bread crusts, raisins, and nuts and put them on the bird feeder.

Discovering Seeds in Fruits and Vegetables

Place several types of fruits or vegetables that contain seeds on a table in the science center. Be sure to have enough so that each child who is interested can have a taste of each food. Talk about how seeds are in some of the foods we eat that come from plants. Explain that plants make seeds so new baby plants can grow.

Cut open each of the foods and see if the children can find the seeds. Talk about which seeds we eat and which ones we do not eat. Let the children taste all the foods and inspect the seeds. Encourage the children to talk about what they are seeing, tasting, and thinking.

Can you find the banana seeds, Tyler?
Yes, they are so tiny!

Extend the Activity

- Have children inspect the seeds in many foods. Try familiar foods, such as peas in pods, strawberries, oranges, grapefruit, grapes, squashes, and melons, as well as more unusual foods such as avocado, okra, eggplant, pomegranate, mango, or papaya.

- Provide magnifying glasses so that children can see the seeds more clearly.

- Have children help remove seeds from each food. Let the seeds dry out a little. Then glue the seeds onto picture cards that show the fruits or vegetables that the seeds came from. Cover the picture and seeds with clear contact paper to make sturdy picture cards. Place these in the science center for children to look at and talk about. Next, make a set of smaller cards that have the seeds without the pictures. See if the children can match the seed

cards to the picture/seed cards. Talk about the foods the seeds came from.

- Put out some vegetables that contain seeds and some that do not for the children to explore. For example, include peas in their pods, corn on the cob, squash, and tomatoes as vegetables with seeds in them and carrots, spinach, lettuce, and radishes as foods without seeds in them. Explain that most vegetable plants do have seeds, but often the seeds are not in the part of the plant that we eat. Encourage the children to taste the foods.

- Bring in some seeds for plants that provide us with vegetables that do not have seeds in them so children can see what the seeds look like. Explain that the flowers of the plants make the seeds to grow the baby plants.

Discovering Seeds in Breads

Bring in several different types of breads that have seeds in them. For example, include rye bread with caraway seeds, bagels with poppy seeds, bread sticks with sesame seeds, sunflower bread with sunflower seeds, and whole wheat bread with wheat berries. See if the children can find the seeds that are in each type of bread and talk about each kind. See what the children can say about how the seeds are the same and how they are different.

The poppy seeds are black. Are any of the other seeds a dark color like the poppy seeds?

Why do you think people put these seeds into the bread?

Allow the children to pull the seeds away from the breads and taste just the seeds alone. Encourage them to taste the seeds with the bread, too. Talk about how all the breads and seeds taste. Explain that many seeds are added to breads for flavoring.

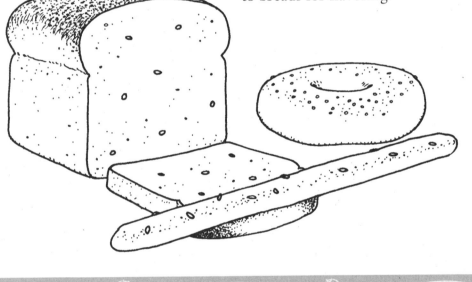

Extend the Activity

- Bring in some containers filled with the different seeds used in making breads. Let the children taste the seeds and talk about them.

- Do a children's cooking activity in which children make their own small loaf of bread, muffin, or pretzel. Provide a choice of seeds for each child to add to the dough.

Children can eat their own baked goods at snack, lunch, or as a special food activity.

- Help the children make a chart to show which seeds they added to their bread, muffin, or pretzel. Talk about which seeds were used most often.

Seeds We Eat Poster

Children can make a poster that shows the seeds we eat. Ask parents and children to help collect seeds, including pumpkin seeds, rice, beans, wheat berries, corn, rye seeds, poppy seeds, and others. Allow children to glue a few of each kind of seed to a large sheet of cardboard or posterboard to make a poster that can be displayed in the science center. The name of each seed can be written on the poster, too.

Talk about the poster with the children. See if they can remember the times they ate the seeds.

These seeds are pumpkin seeds. It says pumpkin *right here next to the seeds. P-U-M-P-K-I-N.*

You brought in these seeds, didn't you, Jeremy?
Where did you get them?

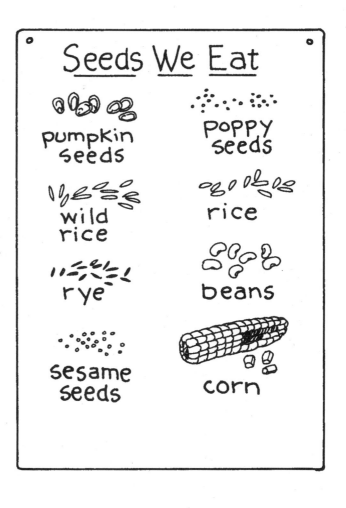

Extend the Activity

- When foods containing seeds are served during meals and snacks, talk about the seeds and show the posters to the children.

- Talk about how seeds are planted to grow new plants.

- Take a nature walk with the children to find any seeds in plants that are growing outdoors. Look for grass seeds or seeds in berries on bushes or other plants. Explain that we do not eat these seeds.

Finding Out About Nuts

Bring in an assortment of nuts in their shells. Show children how the shells can be cracked open to find the meat of the nut. Children will be able to crack open their own peanut shells, but you will have to use a nutcracker to open nuts with hard shells. Allow the children to taste all the different kinds of nuts. Explain that nuts are seeds. See if the children can remember any other seeds they eat. Talk about how the nuts are the same or different, where they grow, and how they taste.

Which nut has the bumpiest shell?

Which nut is the biggest?

Which nut has the softest shell?

Safety Note: Because allergies to nuts and peanuts can sometimes be life threatening, you must be especially aware of children's allergies for this activity. Be sure to double-check with parents about allergies. Also, supervise carefully when young children eat nuts or peanuts to be sure that they do not choke on these foods.

Extend the Activity

- Place a variety of nuts in their shells on the table. See if children can sort the different types of nuts into groups. Tell the children the names of the various nuts. As the children work, talk with them about nuts. Later, crack open the nuts for the children to taste.

- Provide several cooking activities in which children prepare their own recipes that use nuts. For example, children can prepare banana nut muffins, oatmeal with a choice of nuts to add, or peanut butter.

- In the fall, see if you can find some nut trees nearby that have ripe nuts on them. Take a short field trip to visit the trees to see how nuts grow. Compare the nuts that are on the trees to the nuts that come from the store.

From Seeds to Sprouts

Try sprouting some of the seeds that are found in the raw fruits and vegetables the children eat. The children can help you plant them in cups or pots filled with potting soil. Put the pots in a sunny window and water so that the soil is damp but not wet. Talk about what seeds need in order to grow.

Some seeds sprout better than others, so try to use seeds that sprout reasonably well. For example, pumpkin seeds, avocado pits, and grapefruit seeds sprout well: apple seeds require a period of freezing temperature before they will sprout.

Extend the Activity

■ You and the older preschoolers might enjoy trying to sprout lots of different kinds of seeds to see which ones will grow. Be sure to label the seeds so that you will be able to tell what the plants are when they come up.

■ Some foods, such as dried lima beans or peanuts, have tiny plants inside that children can see if they open the seed. Show children how to split the seeds in half to find the tiny plant. It's easiest to open dried lima beans when they have been soaked in water for a day. Talk about how the tiny plant can grow into a bigger plant that then makes new seeds. Talk about how many foods we eat are actually seeds that have tiny plants in them.

■ Sprout some seeds in a plastic jar or cup so that children can see how the tiny plants start to grow out of the seed. Line the jar with a damp paper towel and place the seeds between the jar and towel. Cover the jar with plastic wrap to keep moisture in. Be sure the towel stays damp. Then wait a few days to see if the seeds will sprout. Allow children to look at the sprouted seeds with a magnifying glass. Look at and talk about the new leaves, the stem, and the roots of the new plant.

Changing Foods by Cooking Them

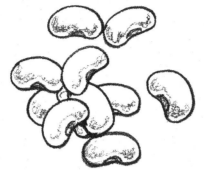

Many of the foods we eat are dried and then cooked for eating. Show children dried beans or peas. Talk about how hard these seeds are when they are dry. Then soak the seeds in water overnight. Allow children who are interested to soak a few seeds of their own. Encourage the children to inspect their seeds to see how they have changed after being soaked. Cook some of the seeds and allow the children to taste them at a meal, snack, or tasting activity. Talk some more about how the seeds change when they are soaked or cooked.

These beans are very soft now that they have been cooked.

Do you remember what they were like yesterday?

Which do you think are easier to eat—the hard beans or the soft beans?

Extend the Activity

- Have the children explore other foods that are hard before being cooked. For example, provide an activity that allows children to discover the differences between cooked and uncooked macaroni, spaghetti, and other dried pastas; rice; potatoes; apples; carrots.

- Arrange for children to discover how some foods change from soft (liquid) to hard (solid) when they are cooked. Let children discover what raw eggs are like and then how raw eggs change when they are cooked. Encourage children to tell about changes they see. Try setting up other cooking activities the children can do in which liquids become solid when they are cooked. Use activities from children's cookbooks that are listed in Appendix G.

Experiencing Different Food Textures

Have several food-tasting activities to help children experience different food textures. For example, one day have children taste crunchy foods, such as carrots, celery, graham crackers, and apples. On another day, have them taste drinks that the children can compare, such as thick fruit shakes, orange juice, and water. Talk about the different textures, sounds, and flavors as the children taste.

Yes, Jasmine, when you chewed that carrot I could hear it crunch. Does the celery make the same noise?

When you drink your shake through the straw it moves very slowly, Jason. What happens when you drink the juice?

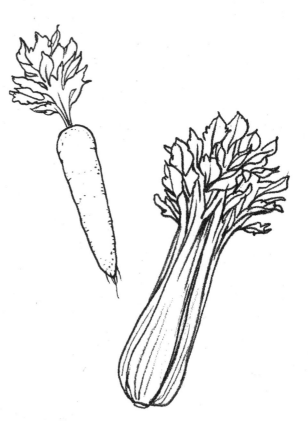

Extend the Activity

- Have children taste raw apple slices, applesauce, baby food applesauce, and apple juice. Talk about the different textures of these apple foods as the children try them.

- Have the children make peanut butter sandwiches using both smooth and crunchy peanut butters on bread, bagels, rice cakes, or crackers. Help the children compare the difference between crunchy

and smooth peanut butter. Talk about which bread was easiest to spread the peanut butter onto.

- Make a chart to show how many children liked the crunchy peanut butter and how many liked the smooth. Help the children count to figure out which was the most popular texture.

Making Juice

Place oranges, grapefruit, and lemons on a table in the science center. Let the children smell each fruit before it is cut open. Then cut open each fruit, one at a time. Let the children smell and taste each fruit. Talk about how juicy the fruits are.

Show the children how the juice comes out when the fruits are squeezed. Let each child try squeezing juice out of a piece of fruit into a cup.

Talk about how hard you have to squeeze to get juice. Look at the pulp that is left after the juice is removed from the fruit. Talk about the seeds that must be removed before drinking the juice.

Bring out a plastic juicer or an electric juicer. Show the children how to make juice from each fruit using the juicers. Note the amount of juice each fruit makes. Let the children taste the juices. Talk about the juices as you make them.

Beth, did you taste the grapefruit juice?
Yes, it's so sour it makes your lips pucker.

How can we get the seeds out of the juice so that we can drink it?

Extend the Activity

- Provide canned, frozen, and fresh juice for the children to taste and compare.

- Provide three or four recipe cards showing each step for making juice.

- Allow children to mix up different juices to make and taste a new juice. Talk about how the taste changes.

- Set up a lemonade-making activity in which the children make their own lemonade by following a recipe.

Discovering How Refrigerators Help Us

Show children a picture of a refrigerator. Ask the children which foods are kept in the refrigerator in their homes. Have children guess what they will find in the refrigerator at the program. Make a short trip to visit the refrigerator and find out what is inside. Talk about how cold things feel when they are in the refrigerator.

See if children can guess what would happen to foods that are left out of the refrigerator for a long time. Then choose a few foods to leave out in the science and math center. Include familiar foods such as milk, a slice of cheese, and raw carrots. Check the foods with the children every day. Compare them with the same foods that were kept in the refrigerator and help children notice the differences. Explain that the refrigerator helps us by keeping food cold so it will not spoil quickly.

What happened to the milk, Aaron?
Yes, it smells bad.

It curdled when it was not kept in the refrigerator. If you drank it now, it would taste sour and might make you sick.

Here's the carrot that was kept cold, and here's the one we left on the table. Are they the same?

Extend the Activity

- During meals or snacks, call children's attention to the foods they eat that are refrigerated. Have them guess which foods came from the refrigerator and which ones did not. Talk about how refrigerated foods are cold.

- Encourage children to tune into which foods must be refrigerated by having them help get foods out and put them away for meals, snacks, and cooking activities.

- Ask parents and children to work together to bring in a list of five things the child eats that are kept in the refrigerator at home. Compare lists to find out what foods are kept in refrigerators.

- Visit a grocery store with the children or ask parents to take their children grocery shopping. Help children discover which foods are refrigerated in grocery stores.

- On a very cold day, place some refrigerated foods outside in a protected, shady spot. Check them with the children to see what happens to them. Try the same thing on a very hot day and place the foods in the sun.

Exploring Frozen Foods

Talk with the children about freezers and take a little trip to visit the freezer. Compare which is colder, the refrigerator or the freezer. Encourage the children to talk about what foods are kept in freezers.

Put a few frozen foods in the science center for children to taste and experience. For example, include frozen peas, frozen strawberries, and some frozen slices of whole wheat bread. Help the children talk about how the frozen foods feel and taste.

Allow the foods to thaw out at room temperature. Then let children taste and experience them again. Talk about how they have changed. See who prefers the frozen foods, who prefers the thawed foods, and who likes both.

Leah liked the frozen peas. Ellen says they were hard like stones. What did you think, Tom?

You liked the thawed bread better than the frozen bread.

Extend the Activity

- Set up activities in which the children prepare frozen foods to eat. For example, allow children to make their own ice cream, frozen bananas, or frozen fruit juice bars. Look for recipes in cookbooks that are listed in Appendix G.

- On a very cold afternoon, put some juice or milk in a covered plastic container. Do not fill it completely. Place it outside in a protected spot. (Each child can put out a small container if you wish.) The next morning, go outside with the children to discover what happened to the milk or juice. Talk about how it changed. Let it thaw a bit and stir it until it becomes slushy. Then everyone can taste and talk some more.

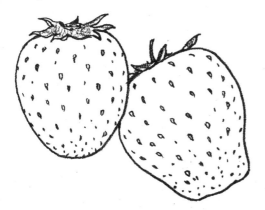

Discovering How Foods Get Moldy

Have some children help you leave some bread out in a damp place until it gets moldy. Show it to the children and tell them about how the mold grew on the bread. Explain that eating food that has mold on it can make you sick.

Help the children think of some foods that might become moldy if left out in a warm, moist place. Try to include moist foods that will grow mold easily, such as cottage cheese, fresh pears, and bread; and foods that are more resistant to mold, such as crackers, uncooked macaroni, and dry cereal. You and the children can check the foods for mold growth every day. See which foods become moldy most quickly.

You're right, Matthew. The cheese is all gray and fuzzy.
Mold grew on the cheese. You don't want to eat it now. It could make you sick.

Do you see mold on the other foods?

Talk about how the moist foods become moldy more easily than the dried foods do, how we store moist foods in refrigerators to keep them from spoiling, and how some foods are dried to keep them from spoiling.

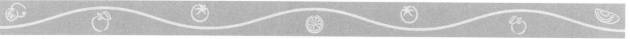

Extend the Activity

- Provide magnifying glasses so that the children can inspect the mold more closely.

- Have children moisten some dried fruit, crackers, and cereal. Place these in a warm, moist place, along with dried fruit, crackers, and cereal that has not been moistened. Check the foods each day with interested children to see which ones grow mold. Talk about how mold likes to grow best on wet foods.

Comparing Fresh, Frozen, and Canned Foods

Have a tasting experience with a food that is in its frozen, canned, and fresh form. For example, provide frozen, canned, and fresh peas for the children to taste. Talk about how the foods are the same and different. Then provide frozen, canned, and fresh carrots to taste. Talk about how they are alike and different, too. See if children remember which of these foods they eat at home.

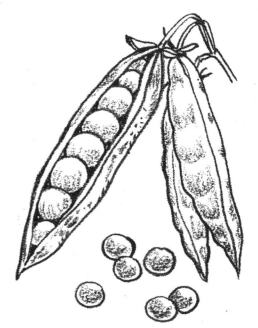

Allow children to cook the foods and then taste them. Find out which ones the children like best.

Jamal liked the frozen peas the best. Gloria says she likes the fresh peas.

What did you think about the vegetables, Beverly?

Extend the Activity

- Provide other foods that are available fresh, frozen, and canned. For example, children can try fresh, frozen, and canned strawberries; fresh and canned tomatoes; fresh, frozen, and canned green beans; and fresh, frozen, and canned corn.

- At meals and snacks, point out which foods are fresh, frozen, or canned. For example, if fish sticks are served, talk about how the fish was frozen and then cooked to be eaten. Have the children cook their own fish sticks for snack one day so they can see the frozen version of the food and see how it changes when it is cooked.

Exploring Fruit and Vegetable Skin

Provide some fruits and vegetables that have skins on them for the children to taste. Have the children help wash the foods. Point out the skins on the foods. Talk about which skins can be eaten and which cannot.

Here's another fruit. That's right, Marcus. It's a banana.

Can you take the skin off the banana?

Do you eat the banana's skin?

How about this pear? Can the pear skin be eaten?

Explain that the skins on fruits and vegetables protect the foods, just as our own skin protects our bodies.

Extend the Activity

- Let the children try foods with and without the skin. For example, if the children are having boiled potatoes at lunch, prepare them with the skin left on. Encourage the children to taste the potatoes with the skin. Then have them try a piece that they have peeled. See what the children have to say about the two different ways to eat the potatoes.

- Have a tasting activity in which the children can try small pieces of broiled or baked chicken with skin. Point out the fat on the skin. Talk about how people do not always eat the fatty skin on chicken. Let the children try a piece of chicken with the skin on. Then let them remove the skin from another piece and taste the chicken without the skin. Encourage the children to talk about how the pieces were the same and different.

- Show how the skins of fruits and vegetables protect the food from growing mold. Make some cuts in foods that have skins, such as apples, pears, bananas, or potatoes. Place cut and uncut foods in a warm, moist place. Check them every day with the children to see which foods get moldy. Point out how mold grows where the skins have been cut because the skins are not protecting the foods.

- Talk about how people have skin that protects different parts of their bodies.

  Our nose has skin covering it. Does your hand have skin? Does your back have skin?

- Talk about how eating fruits and vegetables help skin grow strong. Explain that fruits and vegetables have vitamins that make skin healthy. See if the children can name some fruits and vegetables they eat.

Flowers and Leaves We Eat

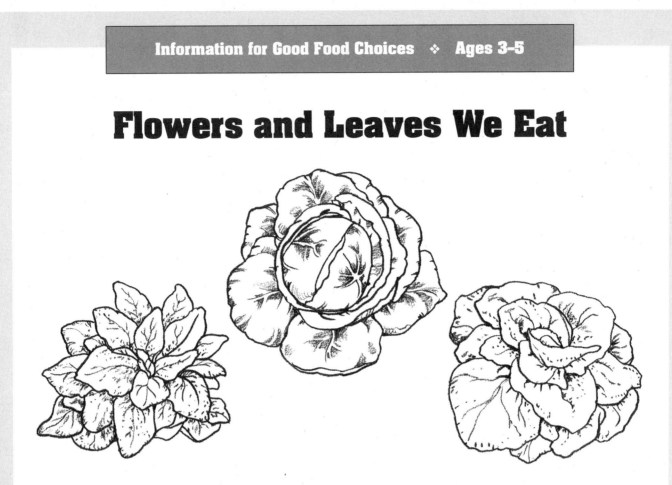

Have a flower- and leaf-tasting activity. To let children taste the flowers of plants, provide raw broccoli and cauliflower. To let children taste leaves of plants, provide different types of lettuce, raw spinach, and raw cabbage. Offer tiny tastes of each to all children. Talk about how these foods are parts of plants.

This vegetable is the flower of the broccoli plant. You can see the tiny flowers that we eat.

Remind children that there are lots of leaves and flowers that cannot be eaten. Tell them that fruits and flowers served at meals and snacks are safe to eat.

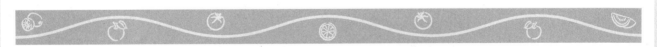

Extend the Activity

■ Help children realize some flowers can be eaten and others cannot. Bring in a few familiar flowers and leaves that people do not use as food and place them on the science table with some flowers and leaves that people do eat. Help the children sort the leaves and flowers into two groups— things we eat and things we do not eat. Allow children to taste the leaves and flowers people do eat.

Discovering How Teeth Work

Provide a few foods of different textures for the children to taste. Offer each child a tiny sample of each. Try to include a soft food such as cottage cheese, a crisp food such as an apple, a bumpy food such as rye bread with caraway seeds, and a tougher food such as celery. As the children chew, talk about how teeth work to grind up the food. Help the children notice how they move their jaws up and down and grind food between their teeth. See if the children can tell you which foods are easier to chew and which require more work.

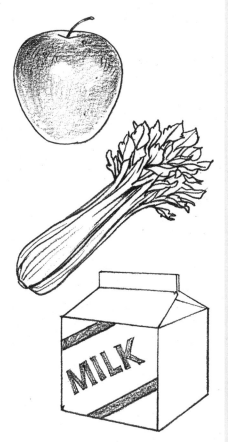

Did you feel your teeth grinding the apple?
Now try this celery. Is it easier to chew or harder to chew?

Remind children that milk products help to build strong teeth. Finish the tasting activity with some milk to drink.

I'm glad we drink milk. It helps our teeth stay strong so they can do all this chewing work.

Talk about how people use the front teeth for biting and the back teeth for chewing as the children eat.

Extend the Activity

- Help the children think about the difference between babies' chewing ability and their own. Show the children a baby doll that has no teeth (or a real baby if a parent can bring in a baby visitor). Talk about what babies can and cannot eat. Help the children compare what babies eat to what three-, four- and five-year-olds are able to manage.

- Have a tasting activity in which children compare baby foods to the regular adult version of several foods. For example, let the children taste pureed pears and raw pear slices, pureed chicken and slices of roasted chicken, and pureed green beans and crisp, steamed green beans. Ask the children which foods they prefer, which needed the most chewing, and which ones babies could eat.

Feeding Happy Tooth Helpful Foods

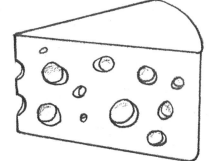

Make a large picture of a tooth on a sheet of cardboard. Give the tooth a happy face with eyes, nose, and a big smiling mouth. Cut out a hole in the mouth that is large enough to insert a picture card. Make a set of food picture cards that the children can fit into the mouth of the tooth face. You will find drawings of the tooth in Appendix H. If you wish, laminate the tooth and picture cards or cover them with clear contact paper.

Introduce Happy Tooth to the children. Talk about how foods made of milk help Happy Tooth grow strong. Let children feed Happy Tooth by putting the food picture cards into its mouth. As the children feed Happy Tooth, help them notice the foods that are made of milk.

What are you feeding Happy Tooth now, Kristi? Oh, it's Swiss cheese. Swiss cheese will help Happy Tooth grow strong because it's made from milk.

Extend the Activity

- Make a large cardboard toothbrush and tube of toothpaste for the children to use to clean Happy Tooth after it is fed. You will find drawings to copy in Appendix H. Talk about how Happy Tooth needs to be brushed after eating. Show the children the toothbrush and remind them to brush Happy Tooth after they have fed it.

- When children are brushing teeth after eating in your program, talk about when Happy Tooth was brushed.

- When children eat foods from the milk group during meals and snacks, remind them how Happy Tooth became stronger from eating these foods.

- Talk about the other foods that the children feed Happy Tooth. Point out the foods that help our bodies to grow strong and healthy in other ways. Help the children notice foods that are high in sugar and point out that Happy Tooth needs brushing even more after eating these foods.

Tasting Foods for Healthy Gums

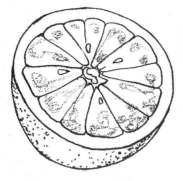 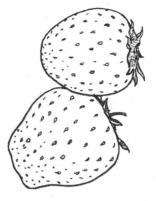

Talk to the children about how our gums help our teeth stay healthy. Allow them to look at their gums in a mirror to see how the gums surround their teeth.

Have a tasting activity in which children taste small samples of the special foods that help keep our gums healthy. Provide samples of foods that are high in vitamin C, such as oranges, grapefruit, and strawberries. As the children taste, let them talk about the foods in many ways—the taste, texture, and smell of the foods, when they have eaten these foods before, where the foods are stored in the supermarket, and so on.

Maya says these foods are sour.

Kendra says they are sweet.

What do you think?

Extend the Activity

■ Set up cooking activities that use foods high in vitamin C. You will find many recipes in the children's cookbooks listed in Appendix G.

■ Place pretend foods that are high in vitamin C in the Pretend Play Center. Include plastic citrus fruits as well as play baby bottles that contain pretend orange juice rather than milk. As children use these props, talk about how these foods help make our bodies healthy.

■ Take a vitamin C trip to the supermarket with the children. Help them find where fresh, frozen, and canned vitamin C foods and drinks are stored.

■ Ask each parent to send in one citrus fruit with their child. Have the children help peel and cut up the fruits and then mix them all together to make a citrus fruit salad for snack.

Growing a Food Garden

If you are interested in gardening and have the time, plant a small garden in a sunny, protected spot where children can see. Plant quick-to-grow vegetables such as radishes and lettuce. If your program operates through the summer, include tomatoes, green beans, and other vegetables that take longer to grow but produce foods that children will enjoy. Be sure to tend the garden well, keeping it weeded and watered as needed so the vegetables will produce well.

Allow any interested children to help you with the garden, but realize that the attention span and abilities of many preschoolers will make it difficult for them to follow through on long-term projects that require many skills, such as gardening. Even though they may not help much, the children will learn lots about how vegetables grow and what it is like to eat vegetables from the garden. You can point out the progress that plants make and the things you do to help the plants grow. Most children will be interested at one time or another even if no one is interested all of the time. A few children might even turn into enthusiastic gardeners.

Do you see a red tomato, Patrick?

Show me! I didn't see one.

Oh, there it is! Shall we pick it for snack?

Let's get the watering can so that we can water the plants.

See how their leaves are droopy? That means they're thirsty.

Extend the Activity

- If you do not have a good place for an outdoor garden, plant small vegetables such as radishes, lettuce, or small tomato plants in containers. Dishpans or large flower pots filled with rich potting soil can be used if kept in a sunny place and watered regularly. You will find a picture recipe for dishpan gardening that children can use in Appendix F.

- Visit a garden at a friend's or child's home so that children can see vegetables growing.

- Read some stories about growing plants. *The Carrot Seed* by Ruth Krauss is a favorite children's book about gardening that should be available through your public library or local bookstore.

Who Ate What for Breakfast Chart

Make a chart to find out about the different foods children in the group eat for breakfast. If you set up the chart on a very big sheet of paper, then the children can help you fill it in.

Begin by having a child identify what he or she ate that morning for breakfast. Write the food at the bottom of the chart and put the child's name above it. Add the names of other children who ate the same thing above the first child's name. As children report eating other foods, add them to the bottom of the chart with names of the children listed above each one.

Help children see which foods were eaten the most or the least by comparing the number of names above each food. Talk about breakfast and why it is important. Tell children that breakfast is eaten to get energy for lots of playing in the morning after not eating all night.

Breakfast Chart

Milk	Eggs	Cereal	Fruit
Lee			
Bob			
Jean		Bob	
Kip		Jean	Lee
Joey	Lee	Joey	Kip
Amy	Kip	Amy	Amy

Extend the Activity

- Children can ask the adults in the program what they ate for breakfast and add the names to the chart.

- Use charts to help children think about many food-related subjects. For example, help children make charts to compare favorite things to drink, favorite vegetables, fruits or other foods, or favorite snacks.

Nutrition Activities for the Science and Math Center

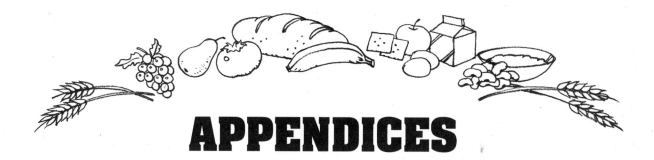

APPENDICES

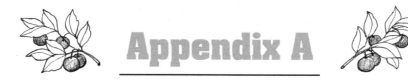

Appendix A

Foods That Can Be Substituted for Foods That Children Do Not Like

Food Substitutions

When a child will not eat a food from one of the groups listed below, you can exchange another food of similar nutritional value if you choose a food from the same group. Remember to limit foods that are high in fats or sugar.

Cereals/Grains/Pasta

bran cereals
cooked cereals
ready-to-eat unsweetened cereals
pasta
brown or white rice

Dried Beans/Peas/Lentils

cooked beans and peas, such as kidney or pinto
beans and split or black-eyed peas
lentils
baked beans

Starchy Vegetables

corn
lima beans
peas
potatoes
winter squash, such as acorn or butternut
yams or sweet potatoes

Bread

bagels
bread sticks
English muffins
hot dog or hamburger buns
pita bread
loaf breads, such as rye, whole wheat, white
rolls

Crackers

animal crackers
graham crackers
matzoh
pretzels
saltine-type crackers
wholewheat crackers with no added fat

Starch Foods That Are Higher in Fat

biscuits
cornbread
butter crackers
french fried potatoes
muffins
pancakes
stuffing
taco shells
waffles
wholewheat crackers with added fat

Lean Meats and Substitutes

beef (round, sirloin, flank steak, tenderloin)
pork (lean ham, Canadian bacon)
veal (any cut except veal cutlets)
poultry without skin (chicken, turkey)
fish (all fresh or frozen, or canned in water)
cottage cheese

Medium Fat Meats and Substitutes

beef (ground beef, rib roast, cubed steak, meatloaf)
pork (chops, roast pork)
lamb (any cut except patties)
poultry with skin (chicken, turkey, ground turkey)
fish (canned in oil and drained)
cheese (skim or part-skim milk cheeses such as
    ricotta or mozzarella)
veal cutlet
egg
tofu
liver

High-Fat Meats and Substitutes

beef (ribs, corned beef)
pork (spare ribs, ground pork, pork sausage)
lamb (patties)
fish (fried)
cheese (all regular cheeses, such as American, blue, Cheddar, Swiss)
luncheon meats (except diet luncheon meats)
sausage, such as Italian or Polish
hot dogs (including beef, pork, turkey and chicken)
peanut butter

Vegetables

asparagus
beans (green, wax, Italian)
bean sprouts
beets
broccoli
Brussels sprouts
cabbage
carrots
cauliflower
celery
cucumbers
eggplant
greens
lettuce
mushrooms
okra
onions
pea pods
peppers
radishes
spinach
summer squash or zucchini
tomatoes
tomato/vegetable juice
turnips
water chestnuts

Fresh, Frozen, and Unsweetened Canned Fruits

apples
unsweetened applesauce
apricots
bananas
berries (blueberries, blackberries, raspberries, strawberries)
cherries
figs
fruit cocktail
grapefruit
grapes
kiwis
mangoes
melons (cantaloupe, watermelon, honeydew)
nectarines
oranges
papayas
peaches
persimmons
pineapples
plums
tangerines

Dried Fruits

apples
apricots
dates
figs
prunes
raisins

Fruit Juices

apple juice or cider
cranberry juice cocktail
grapefruit juice
grape juice
orange juice
pineapple juice
prune juice

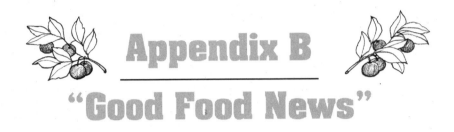

Appendix B

"Good Food News"

GOOD FOOD NEWS

Nutrition Fact

Poorly nourished children do not learn as well as children who eat plenty of healthful foods.

VOLUME 1
NUMBER 1

Encouraging Healthful Eating Habits In Your Child

Parents can do a lot to encourage healthful eating habits in their children that will last the child's lifetime.

The foods served to children should help them to grow strong and healthy. If children fill up on foods that are high in fat and sugar, such as cookies, chips, or sugary drinks, there will be little room left in their stomachs for foods that promote better health. It is best to limit high fat and sugar foods so that they make up the smallest part of what your child can choose to eat.

Sometimes it may seem that your child just does not want to eat any healthful foods. But there are lots of ways to move your child toward healthier eating. Here are a few ideas:

- You can be sure to serve plenty of your child's favorite foods that are not high in sugar and fat.

- You can introduce new foods gradually and encourage but never force your child to taste them.

- You can substitute similar more healthful foods for your child's less healthful favorites. Children who like chips, which are crunchy, may also like crunchy crackers, celery, or low-sugar cereals. Children who like the sweetness of candy will often like toast with low-sugar fruit spread. Children who like ice cream will usually enjoy low-fat frozen yogurt or frozen juice popsicles just as much. Plain cereals with fresh fruit can often replace sugary cereals.

- You can act as a good example by eating foods that are low in fat and sugar.

Exercise!

Along with healthful eating comes exercise. If you have a regular exercise routine, then you are setting a good example for your child. Try to include your child in your exercise whenever you can. Your child might like to take walks, play ball, or rake leaves with you. All of these activities are more healthful than sitting and watching television, and both of you will probably enjoy the active time together.

On The Move!

In your child's preschool program we are working on encouraging healthful habits in your child, too. We can all work together to help your child form the habits for a healthful lifetime.

Talk-About Page

Here are some foods that we serve often in our program. Talk about each one with your child as you look at the pictures together. See if your child can tell you the name of each food and whether he or she likes it or not. Talk about how each tastes and what color it is. Also talk about which of the foods your child eats at home. Go on a food hunt through the kitchen to find out which of these foods are stored at home and where they are kept.

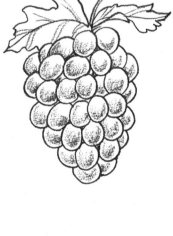

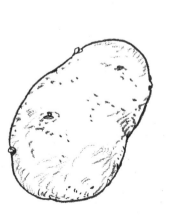

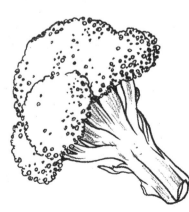

Appendix B: "Good Food News"

GOOD FOOD NEWS

Nutrition Fact

Eating too many foods that contain a lot of fat may lead to health problems later in life.

VOLUME 1 NUMBER 2

Using the Food Guide Pyramid to Make Healthful Food Choices

Are you confused about what types of foods to eat for healthful living? The United States Department of Agriculture has developed an easy system for helping us know which foods to choose. The Food Guide Pyramid, which you will find pictured on the Talk-About Page of this newsletter, helps us remember which foods we should eat most often during a day and which ones to eat less often.

It should be noted that although we should eat more servings of some food groups than of others, no food group is more important than another. For good health we need to eat foods from all the groups shown on the Pyramid.

It may surprise you to find that it is recommended that we

We must take care to limit the fats, oils, and sweets we eat because these foods provide calories but little else.

eat 6–11 servings from the bread, cereal, rice, and pasta food group every day. All of these foods come from grains and supply important nutrients. We get important vitamins, minerals, and fiber from the foods that come from plants: fruits and vegetables.

As you look at the Food Guide Pyramid, you will see that about 4 servings of these types of foods should be eaten each day.

Foods we get from animals should make up a smaller part of what we eat each day. These foods give us protein, calcium, iron, and zinc. Each day we need only about 2–3 servings from the milk, yogurt, and cheese group and 2–3 servings from the meat, poultry, fish, dry beans, eggs, and nuts group.

We must take care to limit the fats, oils, and sweets we eat because these foods provide calories but little else nutritionally. We find fats in foods such as salad dressings, cream, butter, margarine, and foods that have been fried in fat. Sugars are in foods such as candy, soft drinks, and sweet desserts.

In our program we use the Food Guide Pyramid to help us serve your child healthful foods every day.

Talk-About Page

Your child is familiar with the Food Guide Pyramid because we talk about it in our program. Look at the pictures of foods on the pyramid with your child and see which foods he or she can name for you. Talk about the ones you like the best. See which ones your child mentions as favorites.

A Guide to Daily Food Choices

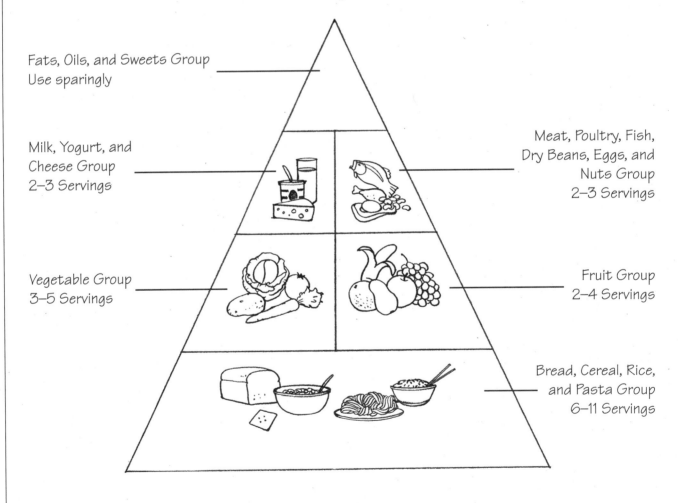

Fats, Oils, and Sweets Group
Use sparingly

Milk, Yogurt, and
Cheese Group
2–3 Servings

Meat, Poultry, Fish,
Dry Beans, Eggs, and
Nuts Group
2–3 Servings

Vegetable Group
3–5 Servings

Fruit Group
2–4 Servings

Bread, Cereal, Rice,
and Pasta Group
6–11 Servings

GOOD FOOD NEWS

Nutrition Fact

Eating sweet, sticky foods too often can lead to tooth decay, especially if tooth brushing does not follow eating these foods.

ENCOURAGING YOUR FAMILY'S GOOD HEALTH

VOLUME 1
NUMBER 3

Choosing Healthful Snacks

Because young children have small stomachs and usually can't eat much at mealtimes, it's important for them to have several small healthful snacks throughout the day. These snacks should satisfy the children's hunger, but not spoil their next meal.

Parents often ask about how to provide healthful snacks that children will eat. Here are some tips for healthful snacks that we follow in our program. You might try following them at home, too.

- Many children prefer crunchy, colorful vegetables such as raw carrots, celery, broccoli, or cauliflower cut up and chilled.

- Children enjoy many fresh fruits. Provide small servings of bananas, peaches, or apples. If you serve grapes, cut them into small pieces so that your child won't choke.

- Favorite snacks from the bread, cereal, rice, and pasta

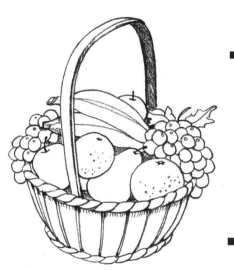

food group include crackers with cheese or peanut butter, graham crackers, or even a little leftover spaghetti. Popcorn without butter is a great snack for older preschoolers, but not for younger children because they can choke on the small pieces.

- Other favorite healthful snacks are frozen juice bars, ice milk, or low-fat frozen

yogurt. Some children like cottage cheese, too.

- Many young children don't like to eat foods that are mixed together. They may not like snacks such as peaches with yogurt, celery with peanut butter, or bananas on cereal, but they will probably eat each of these foods when they are not mixed together.

- Be sure to provide a drink with snacks so that children can take small sips to wash down dry foods as they eat.

Whatever healthful snack you serve, have a few basic rules about where children eat. Don't let children run around while eating because this increases their chance of choking. Sit at a table together, so you can remind your child to chew, swallow, and finish each bite before talking.

Talk-About Page

Here are some favorite snacks we serve at our program. See if your child can tell you the name of each snack, which ones are favorites, and which ones he or she has helped to prepare.

Plan a snack that you and your child can prepare. Then make and eat it together.

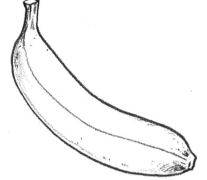

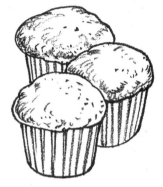

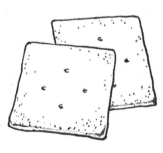

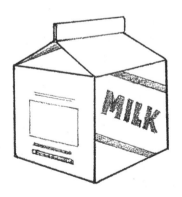

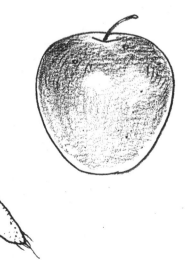

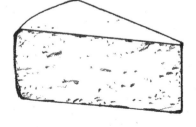

GOOD FOOD NEWS

Nutrition Fact

Children know best how much they want to eat. Suggested serving amounts will meet the needs of the average child, but no child should ever be forced to eat these amounts.

VOLUME 1
NUMBER 4

What To Do If Your Child Won't Eat

Children grow faster at some ages than at others. Three- to five-year-olds usually grow slowly, so they might not be as interested in eating as they were when they were babies. Serving small meals and frequent healthful snacks will help your child get enough to eat each day.

Almost every child will like and dislike certain foods. Some children are more willing than others to try new foods. To be sure that children meet their nutritional needs and build healthy bodies, serve a variety of healthful foods. Then children will have lots of good choices to enjoy.

If your child is a finicky eater, provide regular snacks and meals of healthful foods you know your child likes. Don't pressure your child to eat. Children usually know best how much and what they want to eat. No fuss should be made if children do not want to finish what is on their plate or if they do not like a food. Fussing can cause problems to build up around meals and snacks and things can become much worse. Just wait until the next meal or snack time and serve at least one

> *Serving small meals and frequent healthful snacks will help your child get enough to eat each day.*

healthful food your child enjoys eating.

Preschool children dislike cooked vegetables more than any other food. Some children dislike meats, especially if they are hard to chew. Watch your child to see which cooked vegetables and meats are enjoyable or try a different way of serving a vegetable (mashed, served with cheese on top, shredded, or put into a hamburger).

Children are also more likely to eat foods with child-appeal. Foods with child-appeal are

chewy, soft, or crisp and not tough. Flavors are mild, not too salty or spicy. Like Goldilocks, children like foods that are not too hot, not too cold, but just right. Children like bright, colorful foods, too.

You can try new ways of serving foods to see if your child might prefer a food served in a different way. If your child won't drink milk but likes milkshakes, you can blend milk with a banana and ice. If she or he doesn't drink fruit juices, then try frozen juice cubes that your child has made by pouring juice into ice trays. You can cover the tray with foil and your child can stick a toothpick into each cube as it begins to harden. Making small sandwiches and cutting them into shapes makes them more appealing to some picky eaters. Special cups, dishes, and utensils may also make a difference.

If your child does not eat, appears tired all the time, and lacks energy, an appointment with the doctor may be needed. Otherwise, trust your child to eat when hungry and to eat the healthful foods that are needed for growth.

Talk-About Page

Your child may be more willing to try foods when he or she knows more about them them. Here is a supermarket checklist your child can use on a trip to the grocery store with you. Of course, you don't have to buy all the foods on this checklist. Just use the list as a "food-hunt" activity that will help your child learn about how and where different foods are stored in the supermarket. Have your child look for each item pictured on the list and check off the box as each food is found in the supermarket. Read the words and encourage your child to focus on one picture at a time to make the search go well. Talk about the other foods that are stored near each of the foods on the checklist. Help your child notice whether the foods are stored at hot, cold, or medium temperatures.

Supermarket Checklist

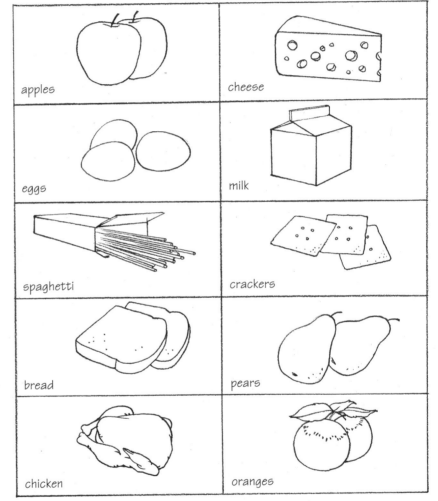

apples

cheese

eggs

milk

spaghetti

crackers

bread

pears

chicken

oranges

Appendix B: "Good Food News"

GOOD FOOD NEWS

Nutrition Fact

Many preschoolers are at risk for iron-deficiency anemia.

Iron Deficiency Anemia

Some preschool children are at risk for iron-deficiency anemia. Iron-deficiency anemia causes children to be tired, less active than others, and unable to learn well. Children with iron-deficiency anemia grow slowly, too.

Serving a variety of healthful foods daily can reduce the risk of having iron-deficiency anemia. Eating foods that are high in iron also helps to prevent the problem.

In the box, foods that are high in iron are listed. Be sure to offer these to your child often. Notice which ones your child enjoys the most and serve them more frequently.

Besides iron, children also need to eat foods that provide vitamin A, vitamin C, B-vitamins, and calcium. All of these are needed for healthy bodies. Vitamin A is needed for healthy

Foods Rich In Iron

- *Lean red meat*
- *Enriched and whole-grain breads and cereals*
- *Dried fruit (peaches, apricots, raisins)*
- *Cooked dried beans (pinto, navy, kidney)*
- *Greens (collard, kale, mustard, spinach, turnip greens)*

skin, good vision, and growth. Vitamin C is needed for healthy gums and to fight infections. Children will get these vitamins if they eat plenty of fruits and vegetables.

B-vitamins are usually found in enriched breakfast cereals and enriched breads. Oatmeal is also a good source of B-vitamins. These vitamins are needed to help our bodies grow normally. Calcium helps build strong bones and teeth. Milk and milk products, such as cheese, cottage cheese, and yogurt supply calcium.

Although many parents give their child a vitamin tablet in the morning, that is not enough. It is important to provide a balanced diet of vitamins in the foods we give our children as well.

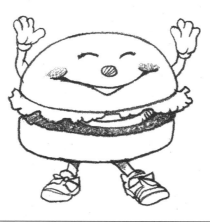

Talk-About Page

These pictures show foods that are high in iron. Talk about the pictures with your child. See which ones he or she can name and which are favorites. Remind your child that these foods help build strong bodies.

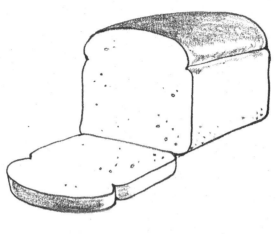

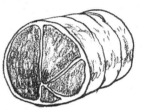

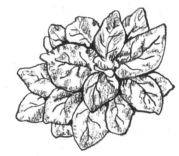

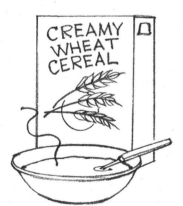

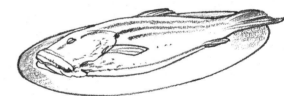

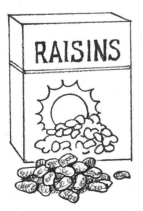

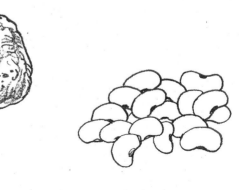

Appendix B: "Good Food News"

GOOD FOOD NEWS

Nutrition Fact

All of the people involved in a child's eating experiences influence the child's eating habits.

ENCOURAGING YOUR FAMILY'S GOOD HEALTH

VOLUME 1 NUMBER 6

Sharing Favorite Foods

Most of us have fond memories of favorite foods we ate when we were children. For some of us it's our grandmother's turkey with stuffing. For others, it's macaroni and cheese. Sometimes our favorite foods are foods of celebration. We ate them for special holidays when we were children, and we serve them to our own families as we celebrate.

Your children are beginning to build their own memories of favorite foods. As you watch them get excited about special meals and foods and listen to them as they ask for a special favorite dish, you realize that they are making memories.

You can share your memories with your children. Perhaps you remember eating snow with syrup or bobbing for apples on Halloween. Maybe you made gingerbread men with your mother and grandmother for Christmas or challah bread for Hannukah. You may have dug sweet potatoes from the garden and mashed them for

Your children are beginning to build their own memories of favorite foods. As you watch them get excited about special meals and listen to them as they ask for a favorite dish you realize that they are making memories.

Thanksgiving dinner. You may remember the first food you ever cooked by yourself or the first time you ate spinach. As you put your child to bed at night or read a story, you can share these memories.

In our program, we are

trying to include memories that children and their families have about food throughout the year. As children write stories or draw pictures about their favorite foods we put them in our Book Center. We have empty food containers of favorite foods in our kitchen area and put pictures of favorite foods on the table for pretend meals.

We would love to have your favorite recipes. If you have favorite food stories or special ways of celebrating that involve food, we would love to hear about them, too, so that we can include food memories from all our families.

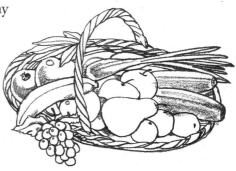

Copyright © Addison-Wesley Publishing Company, Inc.

Appendix B: "Good Food News"

159

Talk-About Page

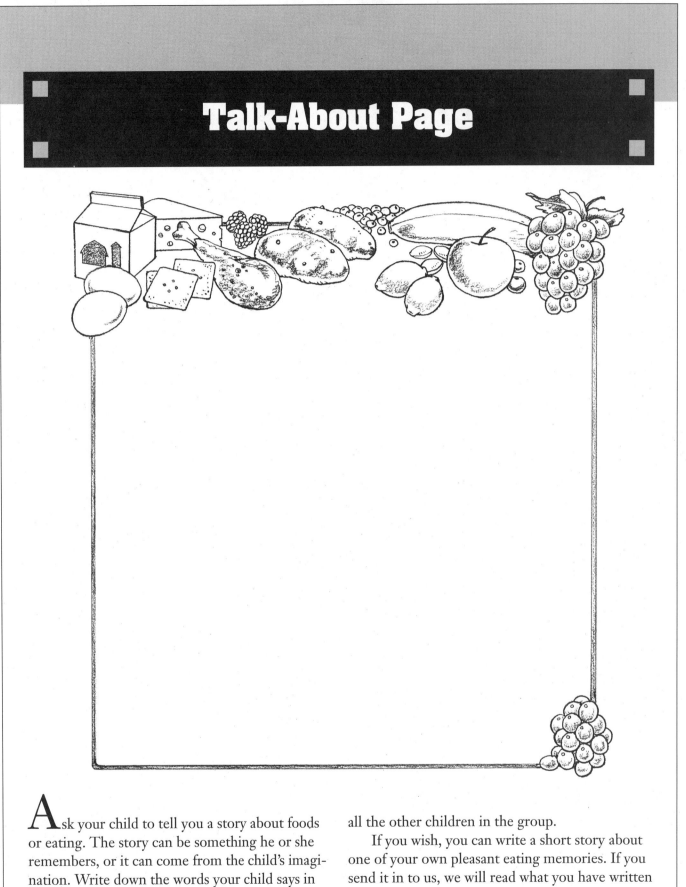

Ask your child to tell you a story about foods or eating. The story can be something he or she remembers, or it can come from the child's imagination. Write down the words your child says in the story space above. Then send the story back to school so that we can read your child's creation to all the other children in the group.

If you wish, you can write a short story about one of your own pleasant eating memories. If you send it in to us, we will read what you have written to your child and his or her friends at school.

Appendix B: "Good Food News"

GOOD FOOD NEWS

Nutrition Fact

Mealtimes should be happy times with little stress and confusion.

VOLUME 1
NUMBER 7

How Children Can Help You at Mealtimes

Mealtimes are busy times for families. Too often everyone is tired, and children are underfoot or in the way. You can turn this into a more pleasant time if you slow things down and let your child learn to help out. Letting your child help at mealtimes will boost his or her feelings of competence, give you some meaningful together-time, and take away some of the pressure. Once you have taught your child what to do and how to do it, mealtimes with your preschooler will become much more enjoyable.

There are many ways your child can help you at mealtime. Children can wash fresh vegetables before you cook them. They can help string beans or shuck corn. They can open boxes of frozen vegetables and get things out of the refrigerator. They can tear the lettuce for a salad and slice cucumbers or grate carrots.

Your child can help set the table. Perhaps you and your child can plan a special decoration for the center of the table once a week, either flowers or some-

> *Letting your child help at mealtimes will boost his or her feelings of competence, give you some meaningful together-time, and take away some of the pressure.*

thing your child has made. If you have several children, they can take turns decorating the table.

At our program we serve some foods family style, so that children can help themselves and can get seconds if they like. We have a small pitcher so that the children can pour milk or juice and can get more if they are thirsty. A small pitcher makes it easier for a young child to pour without spilling, but we keep extra napkins, sponges, or paper

towels on hand just in case. Pouring is harder than we remember, and it takes lots of practice! At home, your child can serve his or her own foods, too.

Children can also help with cleanup. They can take dirty dishes from the table to the sink (using a plastic dishpan), and they can rinse the dishes so that you can wash them or put them in the dishwasher. Of course, if you are using your special dishes you might ask your child to bring the dirty silverware instead. Children can also wipe the table after it has been cleared. A small damp sponge makes this easier.

You and your child might want to try cooking a simple meal together. Children like to make French toast or help you scramble some eggs. They can mix up some orange juice or bring you things you need. This is a good time for your child to try new foods, since children are more likely to taste foods they have cooked themselves.

In our program children prepare some of their own foods. One of our favorite recipes is a Chinese chicken noodle soup from *Cook and Learn* by Beverly Veitch and Thelma Harms, published by Addison-Wesley Publishing Company. Here is the recipe we followed. Talk about the recipe with your child. See if he or she can tell you about each step.

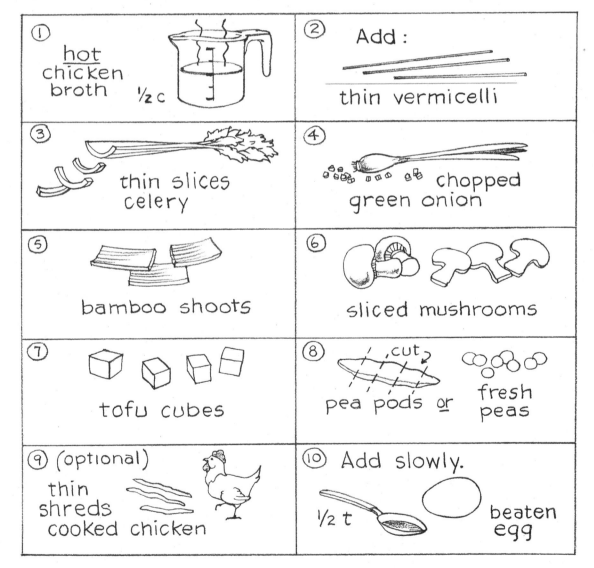

① <u>hot</u> chicken broth ½ c	② Add: ——————— thin vermicelli
③ thin slices celery	④ chopped green onion
⑤ bamboo shoots	⑥ sliced mushrooms
⑦ tofu cubes	⑧ cut→ pea pods or fresh peas
⑨ (optional) thin shreds cooked chicken	⑩ Add slowly. ½ t beaten egg

GOOD FOOD NEWS

Nutrition Fact

Frequent and regular handwashing is one of the best ways to cut down on the spread of germs and illness.

ENCOURAGING YOUR FAMILY'S GOOD HEALTH

VOLUME 1 NUMBER 8

Making Handwashing a Habit

Experts have found that one of the best ways to cut down on the spread of germs and illnesses is by washing hands often as a regular part of each day. In our program we make sure that children wash hands when needed—before eating meals and snacks, before helping to prepare foods or set the table, and after they use the toilet or wipe their nose. Adults are sure to wash their hands at these times, too.

Parents and other family members can help children make regular handwashing a habit at home. For proper handwashing, children need to be able to reach the water, soap, and towels safely and easily. Children should use soap and running water, rubbing their hands together. They should be taught to wash the front and back of hands, to wash between fingers and under fingernails. After washing, they should be

When other family members set a good example, it is easier for the child to make handwashing a habit.

taught how to rinse and then dry hands on a clean towel. Your child may need to be reminded to turn off the water and to manage hot water safely, too.

If your child forgets to wash hands, remind him to do so. Show him how to wash his hands thoroughly if he doesn't do it on his own. Tell him why it's important to wash his hands.

Make sure that all family members wash their hands before meals or before meal preparation, too. When other family members set a good example, it is easier for the child to make handwashing a habit.

The Talk-About Page shows the steps for handwashing that we use at our program. See if your child can talk about what the pictures tell him to do. You can cut out the pictures, mix them up, and then see if your child can put them in the right order again.

Talk-About Page

These are the steps of handwashing that your child has learned while in our program. Look at the pictures and see if your child can tell you about each one.

Cut out the pictures and mix them up. Then see if your child can put them back in the correct order and tell you which comes first, second, third, and so on.

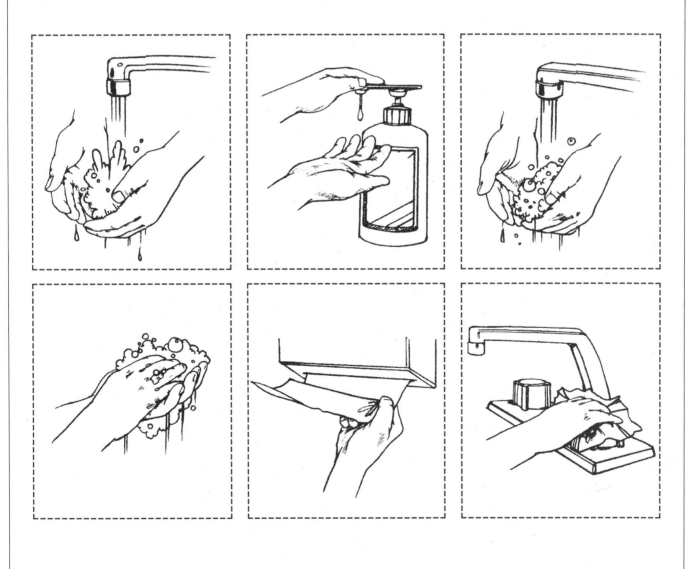

Appendix B: "Good Food News"

GOOD FOOD NEWS

Nutrition Fact

Teachers and parents should work together to encourage good eating habits at home and in the early childhood program.

Ways Parents Can Help With Nutrition Education At School

Every day in early childhood programs and at home, children's experiences with foods are helping to form long-lasting eating habits. Parents have the major influence at home; the teaching staff has the major influence at school. The closer these important adults work together, the better it is for the child.

We need you to work with us as partners in nutrition education. There are many ways you and other parents can help us, depending on the time you have and the things you feel most comfortable doing.

Here are some ideas about how you can help:

- Visit our program and eat lunch with your child. Later, talk about the foods that were served.

- Donate ingredients or utensils to be used in cooking

> *We need parents to work with us as partners in nutrition education.*

activities. If you are an organizer, you might even plan a "Cooking Shower" to equip your child's classroom for cooking.

- Help with a classroom cooking activity or teach children a nutrition-related game. Even a half hour can be very productive if the staff can plan ahead with you.

- Help teachers take children

on a nutrition-related field trip. You might suggest a good place for children to visit, help plan the trip, or go with the class and help with transportation, supervision, and talking about what the children see and do.

- Collect clean, empty containers that healthful foods were in. Bring them in so that they can be used as children play house or store. Be sure containers are safe—no glass or sharp edges.

Whatever way you choose to help with your child's nutrition education, let our staff know you're interested, so that a plan to involve you can be worked out.

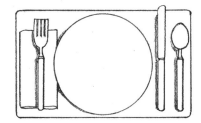

Talk-About Page

This is a recipe for "dishpan gardening" that we have used in our classroom. See if your child can look at the pictures and tell you a little about each one. If you have a garden or many plants at your house, let your child help take care of them. Point out any plants that are grown as food.

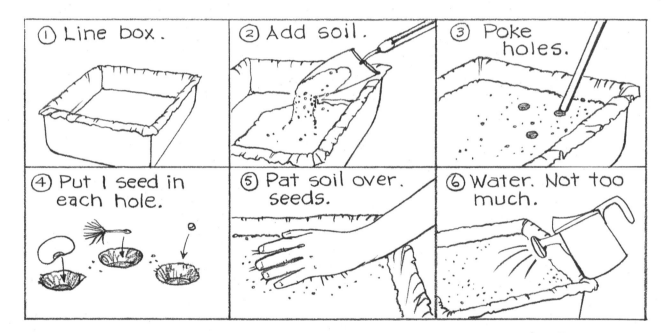

① Line box.

② Add soil.

③ Poke holes.

④ Put 1 seed in each hole.

⑤ Pat soil over seeds.

⑥ Water. Not too much.

Appendix B: "Good Food News"

GOOD FOOD NEWS

Nutrition Fact
Children are more likely to accept a new food when they have learned about it before trying it.

Choosing Books and Games for Children

As concerned parents and teachers, we encourage children to try new foods and develop good food habits. But we must be aware of the messages about food that children get daily from the television they watch, the books they look at, and the games they play. Many of those messages are not good for children because they glorify candy, cereals containing a lot of sugar, and high-calorie snack foods that do not provide much nutrition.

By selecting books and games that make foods interesting, we can give the right ideas about foods a chance to influence our children. Here are a few such books you can get at the library:

The Very Hungry Caterpillar by Eric Carle. William Collins and World Publishing Inc., Cleveland, OH.

Bread and Jam for Frances by Russell Hoban. Scholastic Book Services, NY.

The Carrot Seed by Ruth Krauss. Scholastic Book Services, NY.

> *We must be aware of the messages about food that children get daily from the television they watch, the books they look at, and the games they play.*

Blueberries for Sal by Robert McCloskey. Penguin Books, NY.

Mr. Rabbit and the Lovely Present by Charlotte Zolotow. Harper and Row Publishers, NY.

When you read these books with your child, point out what is being eaten and why it's good to eat that food. If possible, have the same or a similar food as a snack or part of the meal that day.

Look at the games your child already has. If they contain food ideas, do they reinforce good eating habits or, like some commercial games, do they emphasize less healthful foods? When you select new games, consider the food-related ideas these games promote and choose those that instill good ideas. The game on the Talk-About Page is one you can make at home for your child. Ask the teachers for more suggestions for books and games that give children the right ideas about food.

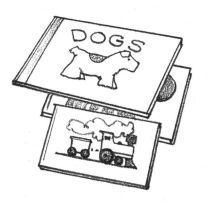

Jump to Strong Teeth and Gums

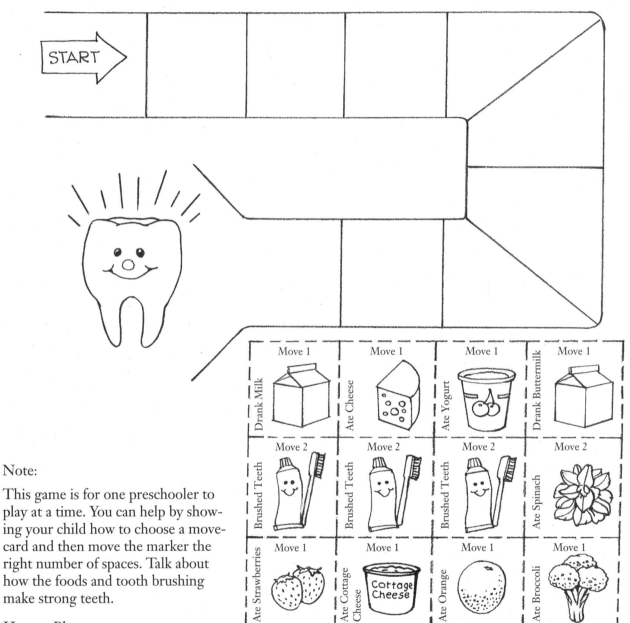

START

Move 1 Drank Milk	Move 1 Ate Cheese	Move 1 Ate Yogurt	Move 1 Drank Buttermilk
Move 2 Brushed Teeth	Move 2 Brushed Teeth	Move 2 Brushed Teeth	Move 2 Ate Spinach
Move 1 Ate Strawberries	Move 1 Ate Cottage Cheese	Move 1 Ate Orange	Move 1 Ate Broccoli

Note:

This game is for one preschooler to play at a time. You can help by showing your child how to choose a move-card and then move the marker the right number of spaces. Talk about how the foods and tooth brushing make strong teeth.

How to Play

1. Use a button or pebble for your child's marker.

2. Cut out move-cards. Shuffle and place face down.

3. Choose a move-card. Child can talk about food picture or say what he did to build strong teeth and gums. Move the marker the correct number of spaces.

4. Child can play until finished. Reshuffle, turn cards face down, and play again.

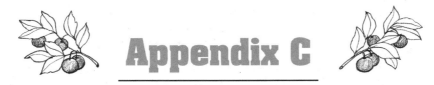

Appendix C

Masters for Food Picture Matching Games

- Directions: Copy, color, and cut out to make food picture cards.

- Note: These pictures are not meant to be coloring book pages for children. Children are most creative when they draw or design their own artwork rather than just coloring an adult's drawing. Adults may color these pictures to make them more appealing to children when used in an activity.

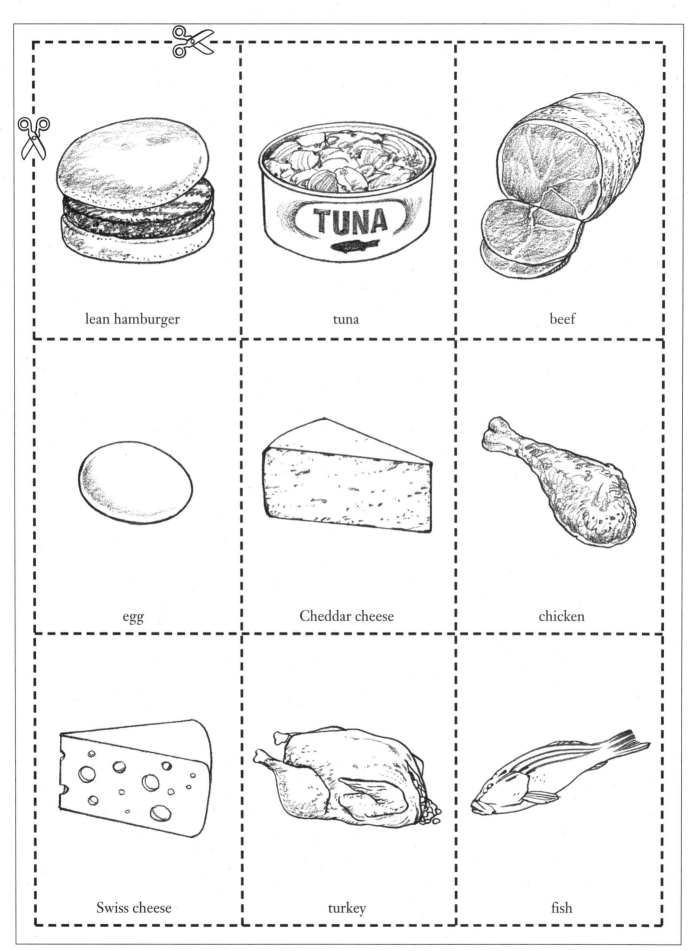

lean hamburger

tuna

beef

egg

Cheddar cheese

chicken

Swiss cheese

turkey

fish

Appendix C: Picture Matching Game

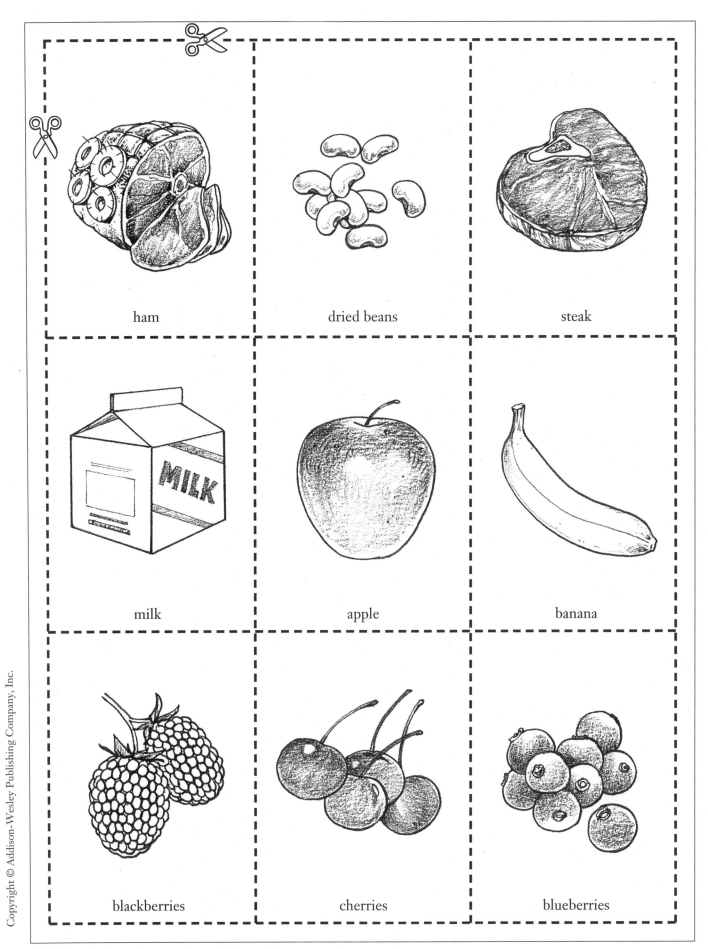

ham

dried beans

steak

milk

apple

banana

blackberries

cherries

blueberries

Appendix C: Picture Matching Game

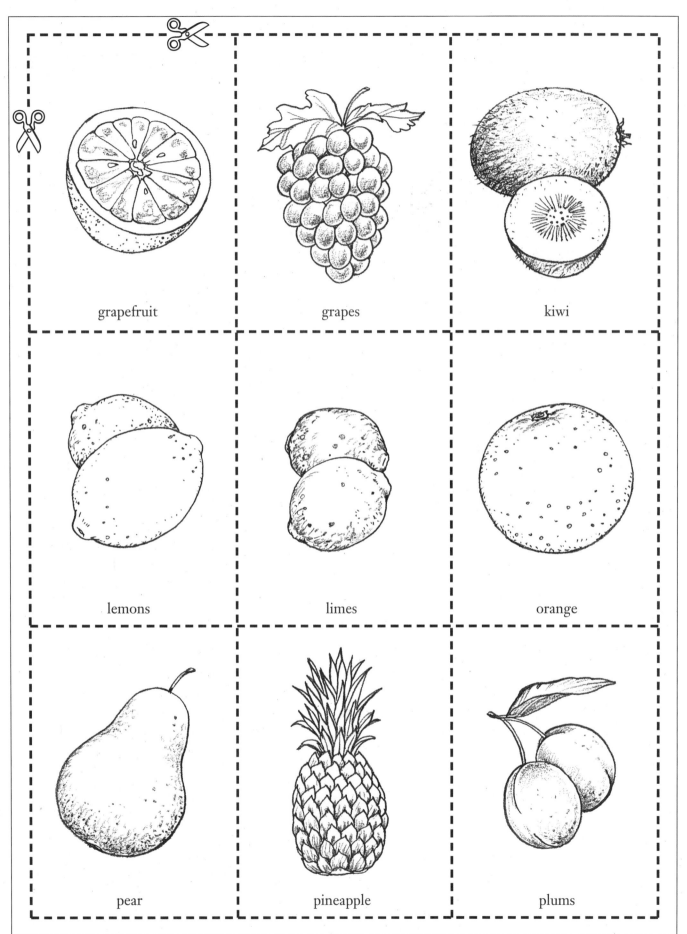

grapefruit

grapes

kiwi

lemons

limes

orange

pear

pineapple

plums

Appendix C: Picture Matching Game

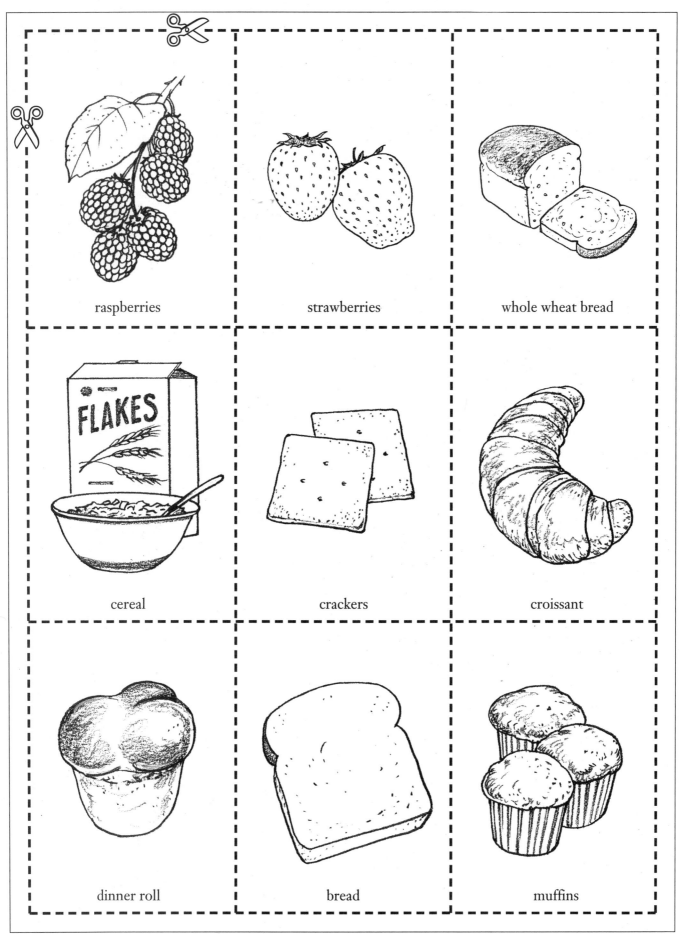

raspberries

strawberries

whole wheat bread

cereal

crackers

croissant

dinner roll

bread

muffins

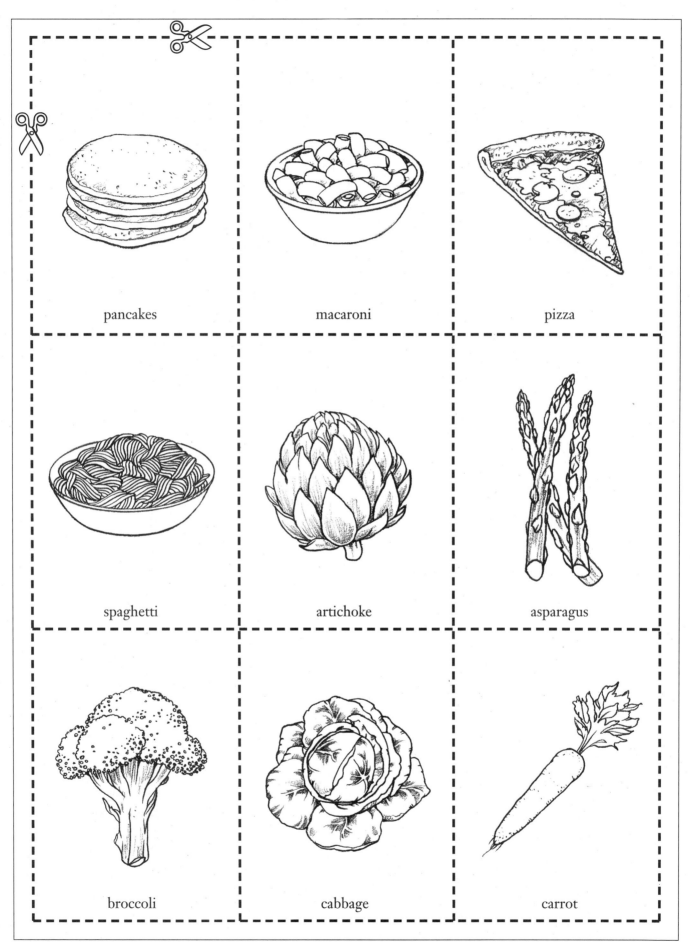

pancakes

macaroni

pizza

spaghetti

artichoke

asparagus

broccoli

cabbage

carrot

Appendix C: Picture Matching Game

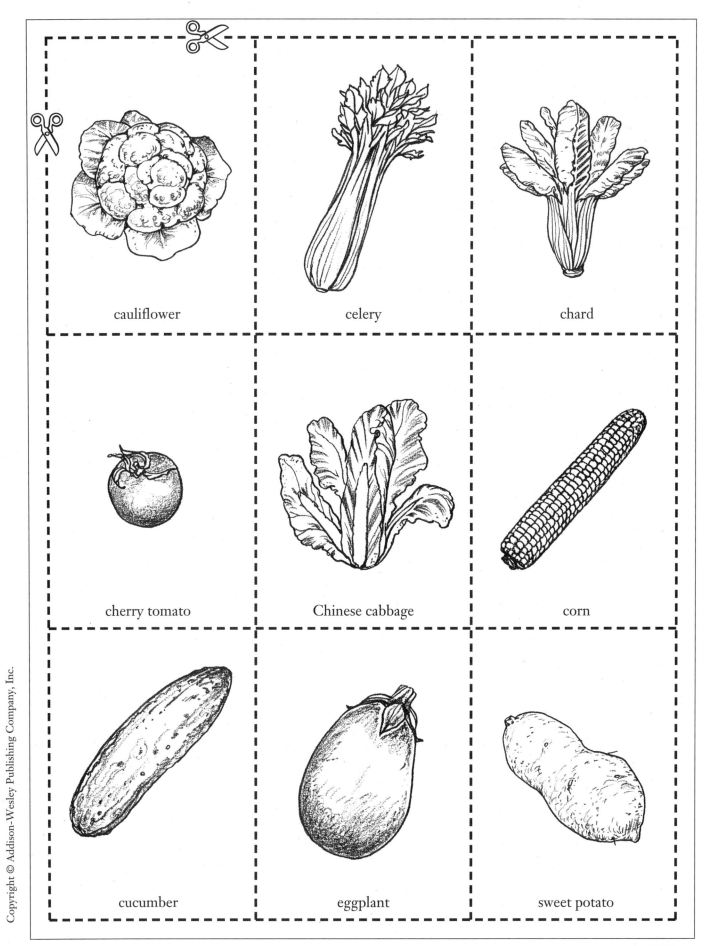

cauliflower

celery

chard

cherry tomato

Chinese cabbage

corn

cucumber

eggplant

sweet potato

Appendix C: Picture Matching Game

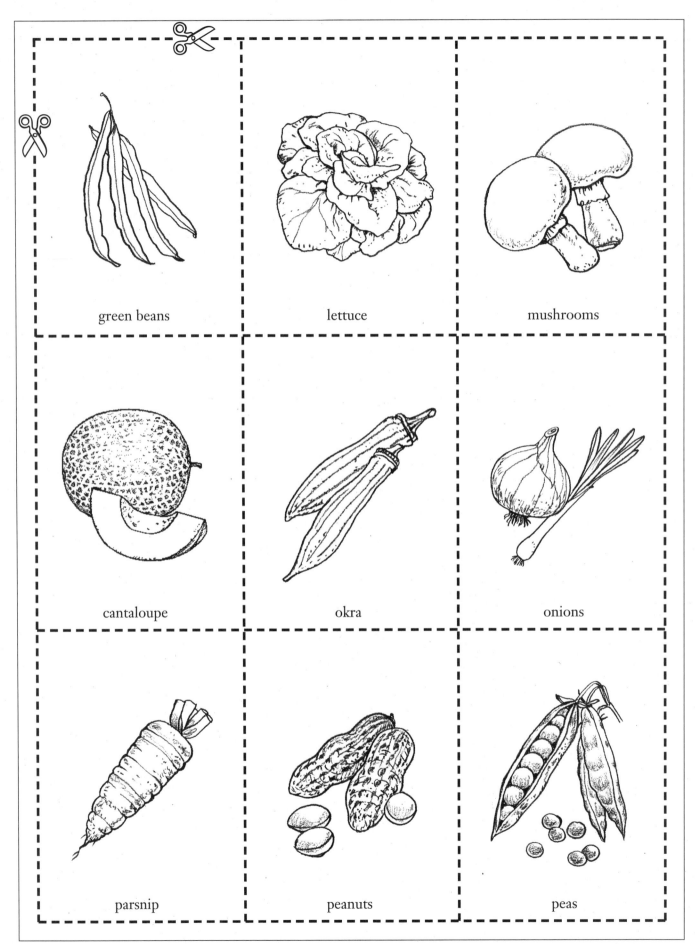

green beans

lettuce

mushrooms

cantaloupe

okra

onions

parsnip

peanuts

peas

Appendix C: Picture Matching Game

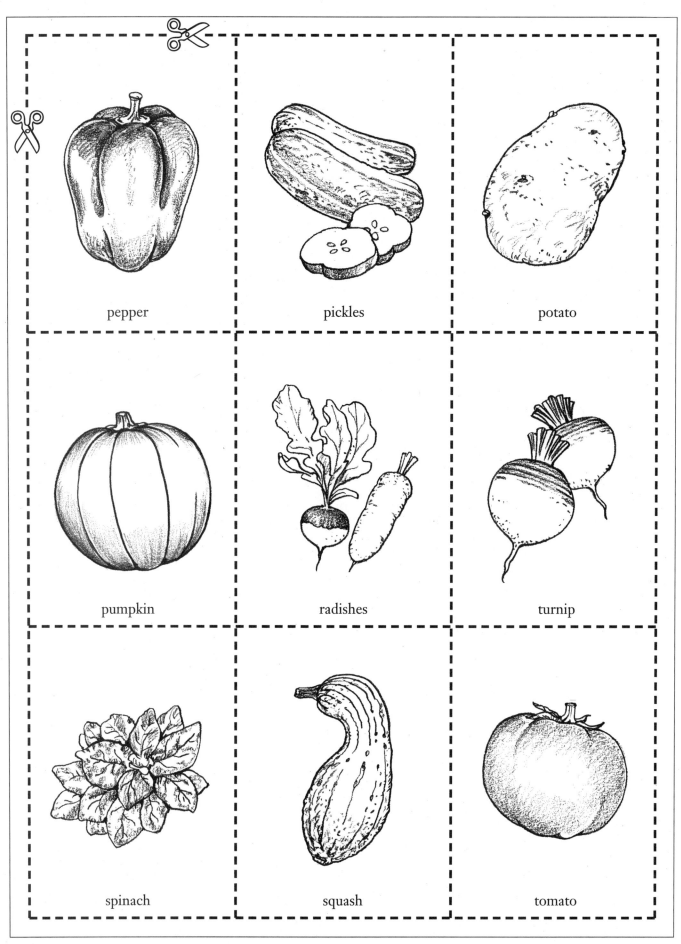

pepper

pickles

potato

pumpkin

radishes

turnip

spinach

squash

tomato

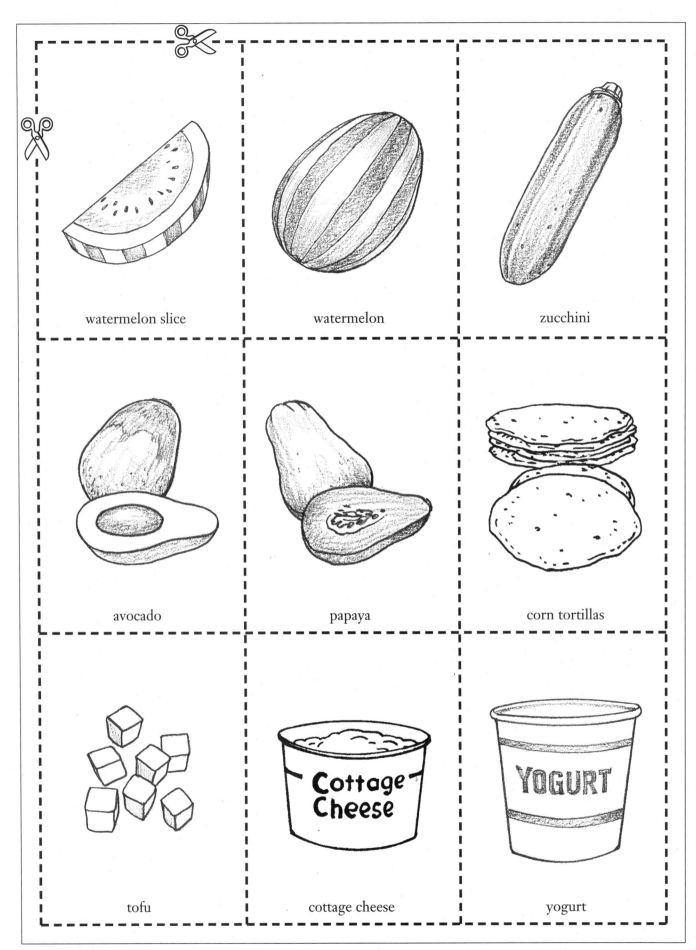

watermelon slice

watermelon

zucchini

avocado

papaya

corn tortillas

tofu

Cottage Cheese

cottage cheese

YOGURT

yogurt

Appendix C: Picture Matching Game

Appendix D:

Masters for How Foods Help Us Matching Games

Directions: Each large picture shows a part of the body and some of the foods that help it. Children match a set of individual food pictures to the pictures on this page.

1. Protect the large pictures by gluing to cardboard, laminating, or covering with clear contact paper. You can color the pictures to make them more appealing to children.

2. Cut out the individual food picture cards. Glue them to cardboard and laminate or cover with clear contact paper.

3. Show children how to match each picture card to the same food on the larger card.

Note: These pictures are not meant to be coloring book pages for children. Children are most creative when they draw or design their own artwork rather than just coloring an adult's drawing. Adults may color these pictures to make them more appealing to children when used in an activity.

These foods have calcium that helps us have strong bones and teeth.

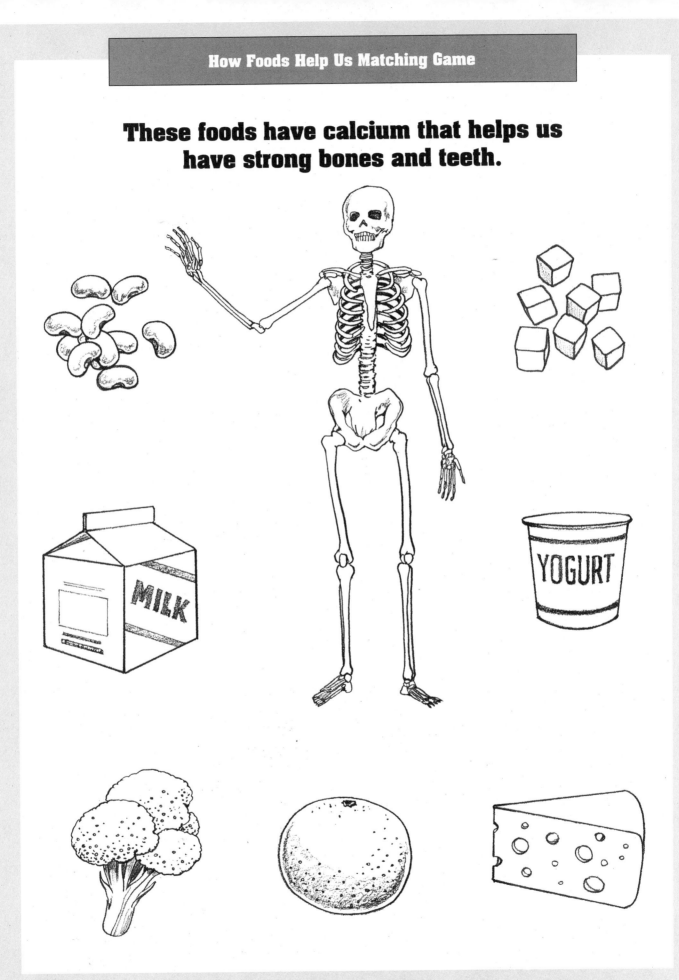

Appendix D: How Foods Help Us Games

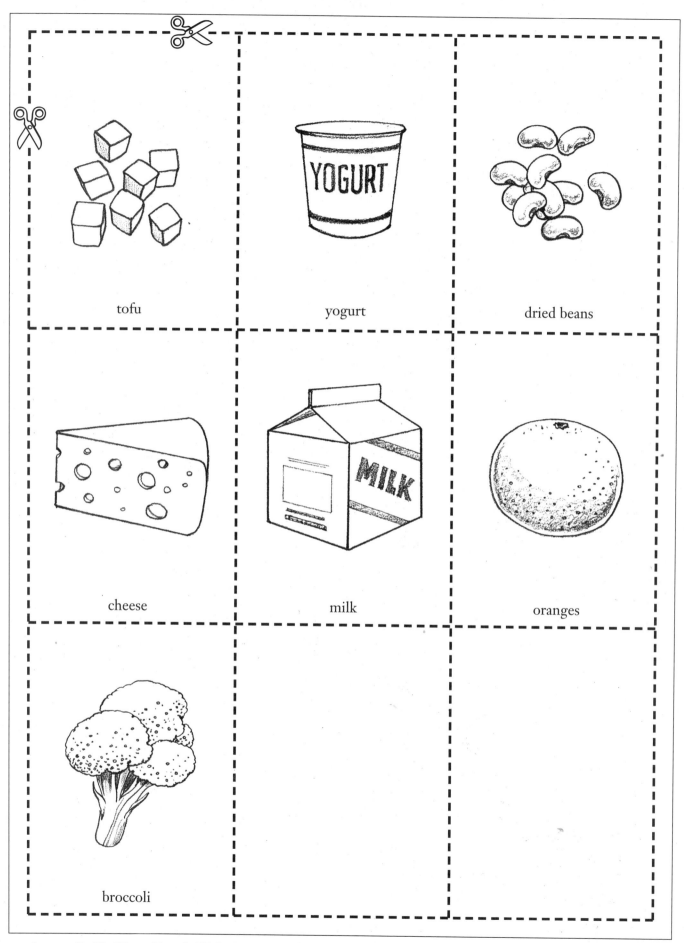

tofu

yogurt

dried beans

cheese

milk

oranges

broccoli

Appendix D: How Foods Help Us Games

These foods help us have strong blood for lots of energy.

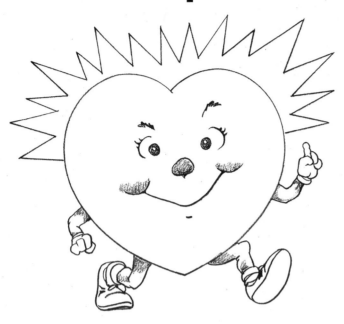

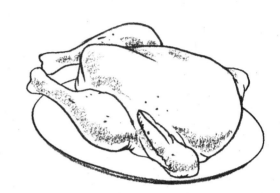

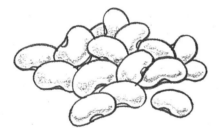

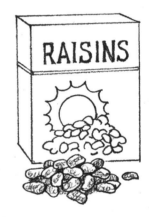

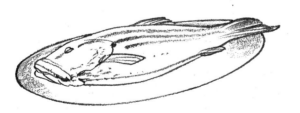

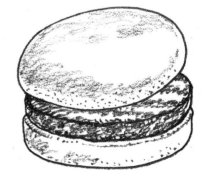

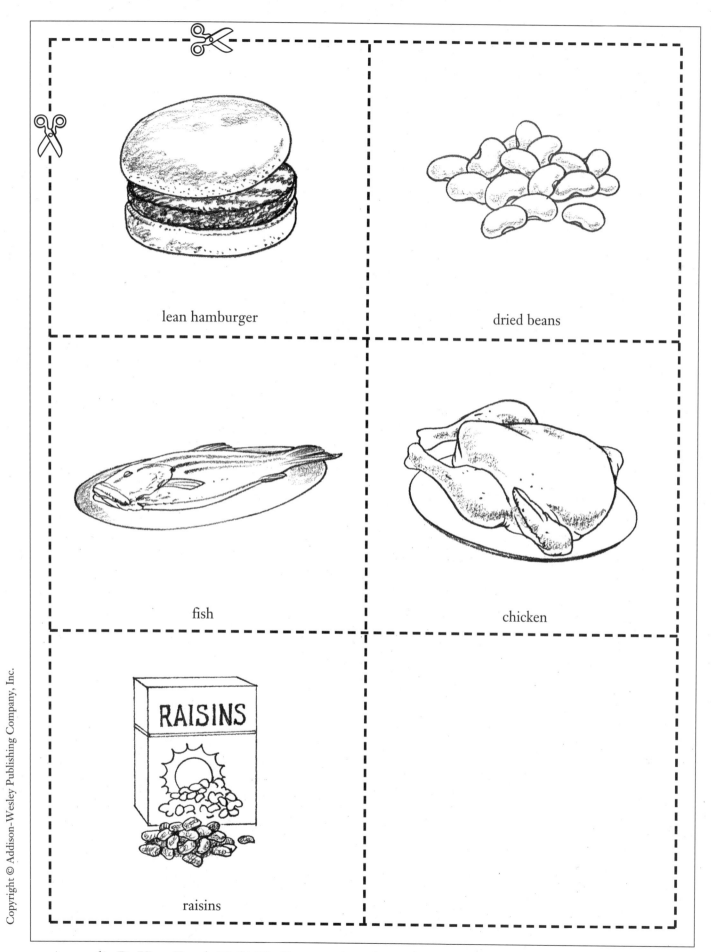

lean hamburger

dried beans

fish

chicken

RAISINS

raisins

These foods help us have healthy eyes.

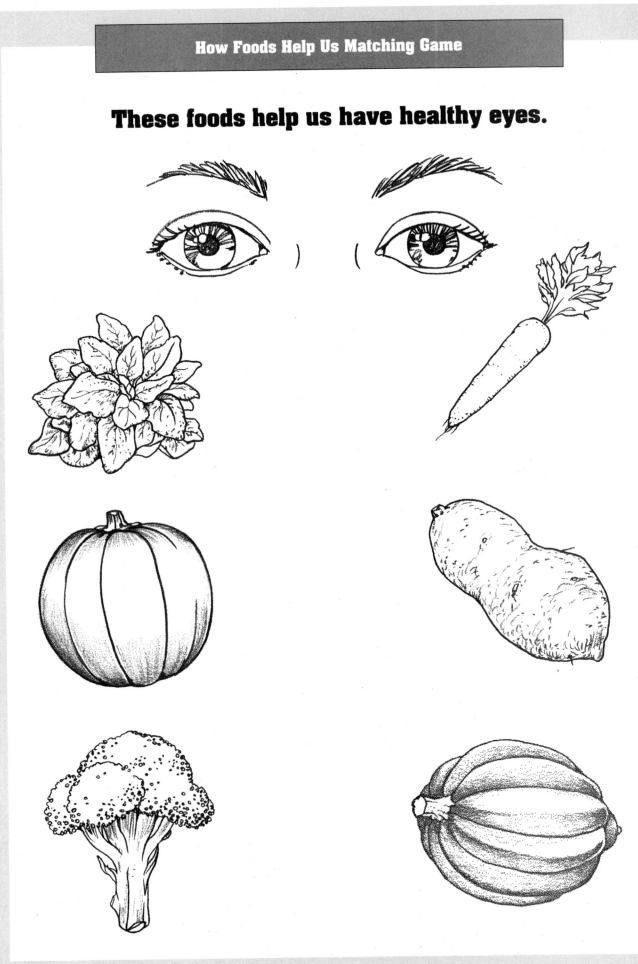

Appendix D: How Foods Help Us Games

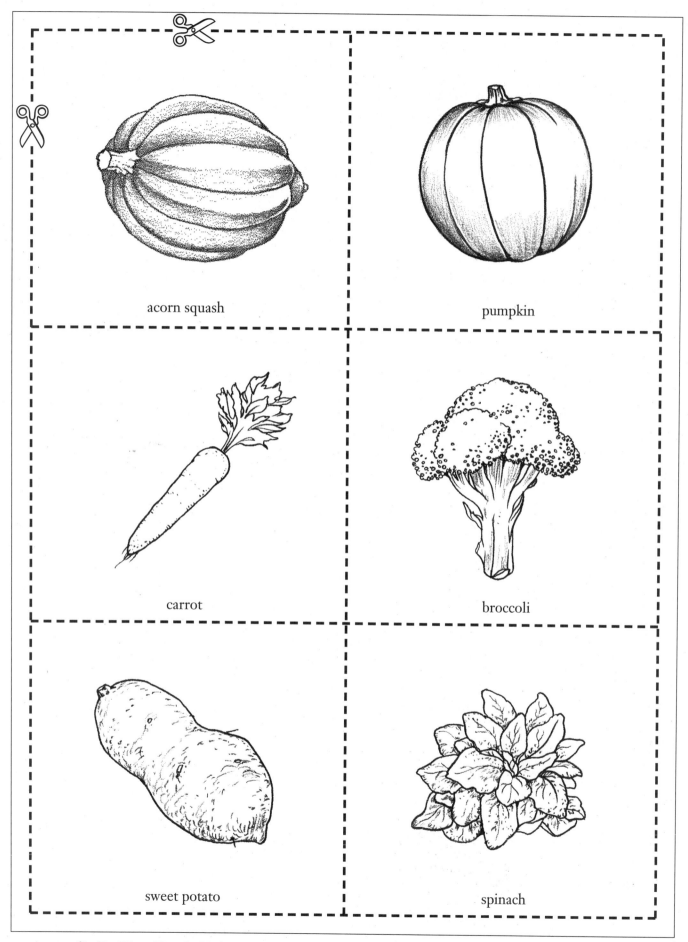

acorn squash

pumpkin

carrot

broccoli

sweet potato

spinach

These foods help us have strong gums and help keep us from getting sick.

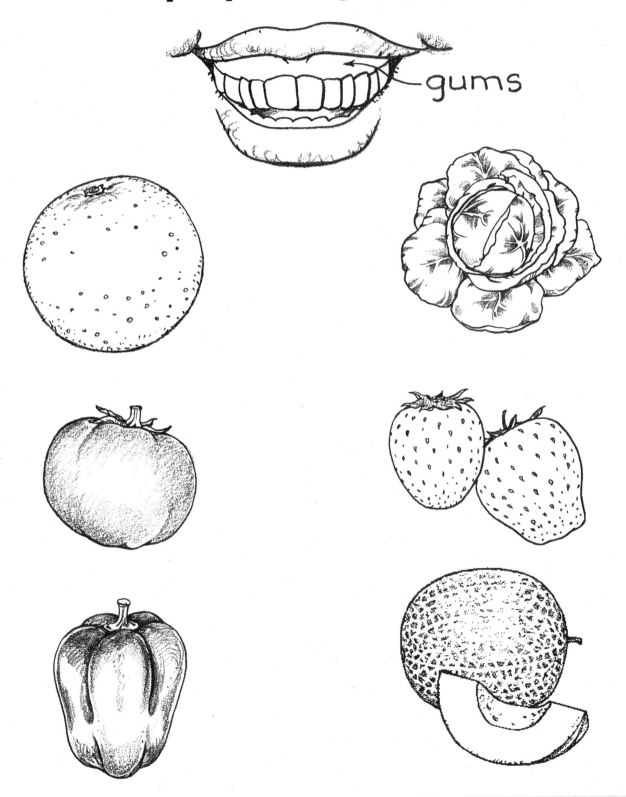

gums

Appendix D: How Foods Help Us Games

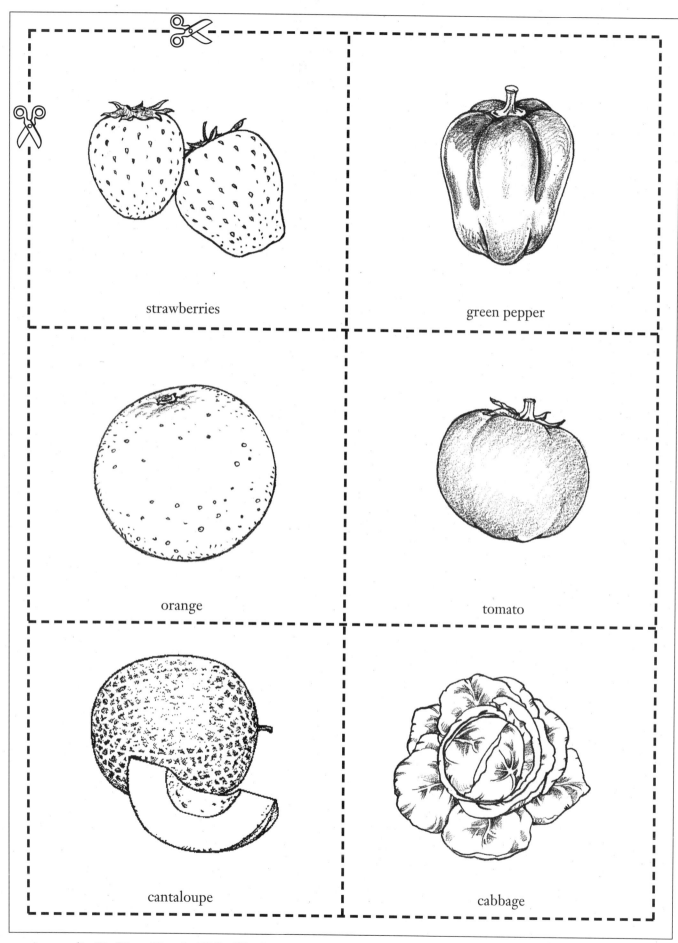

strawberries

green pepper

orange

tomato

cantaloupe

cabbage

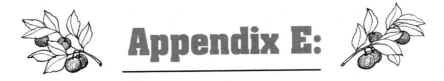

Appendix E:
Resources for Nutrition Information

Resources for Nutrition Information

The following list of organizations can provide free or low-cost food and nutrition materials. We suggest that you make your requests in advance, since you will usually need to obtain publication lists and order forms before you can actually order materials.

Professional/Volunteer Organizations

American Dental Association
211 East Chicago Avenue
Chicago, IL 60611
1-800-621-8099

American Diabetes Association
National Service Center
1660 Duke Street
P.O. Box 25757
Alexandria, VA 22314

American Dietetic Association
216 West Jackson Blvd., Suite 800
Chicago, IL 60606
1-800-877-0877

American Heart Association, National Center
7320 Greenville Avenue
Dallas, TX 75231

American Medical Association
Nutrition Information Service
515 North State Street
Chicago, IL 60610
312-645-4818

American Public Health Association
1015 Fifteenth Street, NW
Washington, DC 20005
202-789-5600

American Red Cross
18th and E Street
Washington, DC 20006

American School Food Service
1600 Duke Street, 7th Floor
Alexandria, VA 22314-3436
1-800-877-8822

National Association for the
    Education of Young Children
1509 Sixteenth Street, NW
Washington, DC 20036-1426
1-800-424-2460

National Cancer Institute
Office of Cancer Communication
Building 31, Room 104-18
Bethesda, MD 22025

Government and State Agencies

Center for Science in the Public Interest
1875 Connecticut Avenue, NW
Suite 300
Washington, DC 20009
202-332-9110

Community Nutrition Institute
2001 S Street, NW
Washington, DC 20009
202-462-4700

Food and Drug Administration
Center for Food Safety and Nutrition
200 C Street, SW, FB-8
Washington, DC 20204
202-245-8850

Food and Nutrition Information Center
National Agriculture Library
10301 Baltimore Blvd., Room 304
Beltsville, MD 20705
301-344-3719

National Health Information Clearinghouse
P.O. Box 1133
Washington, DC 20013
1-800-336-4797

National Maternal and Child Health
  Clearinghouse
3520 Prospect Street, NW
Washington, DC 20057

President's Council on Physical Fitness
  and Sports
450 Fifth Street, NW, Suite 7103
Washington, DC 20001
202-272-3427

U.S. Department of Agriculture
Human Nutrition Information Service
6505 Belcrest Road, Room 360
Hyattsville, MD 20782
301-436-7725

U.S. Department of Agriculture
Office of Governmental and Public Affairs
Washington, DC 20250

U.S. Department of Health and
  Human Services
National Institute of Health and
Human Services
9000 Rockville Pike
Bethesda, MD 20014

U.S. Department of Health and
  Human Services
Public Health Services
5600 Fishers Lane
Rockville, NC 20857

U.S. Government Printing Office
Superintendent of Documents
Washington, DC 20402-9325

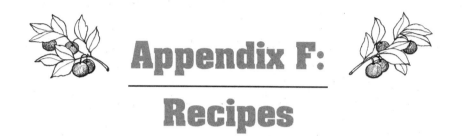

Appendix F:
Recipes

Recipe for Play Dough

Play Dough for One Child to Make

1. The child measures and pours into a medium bowl:

   1 cup flour

   1/2 cup salt

   1/8 cup oil

   1/4 cup water

   few drops of food coloring

2. The child stirs with a large spoon until the ingredients become easier to mix and the food coloring is well-mixed with the other ingredients. An adult can help the child add more water or flour, a tablespoon at a time, until the mixture is firm, not too wet, and sticks together.

3. The child kneads and squeezes the mixture until a smooth dough is made.

Play Dough for a Group of Children

1. Measure and pour into a large bowl:

   4 cups flour

   2 cups salt

   1/2 cup oil

   1 cup water

   1 teaspoon food coloring

2. Stir with a large spoon until the ingredients become easier to mix and the food coloring is well-mixed with the other ingredients. Add more water or flour, a tablespoon at a time, until the mixture is firm, not too wet, and sticks together.

3. Knead and squeeze the mixture until a smooth dough is made.

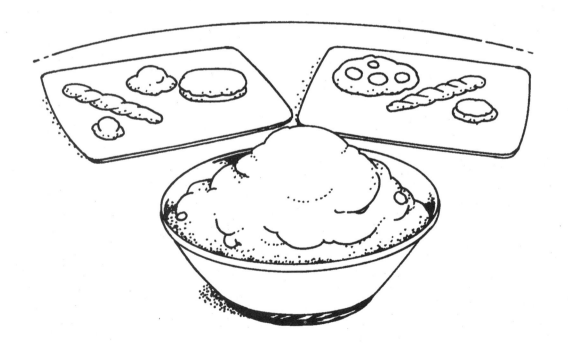

Appendix F: Recipes

Recipe for Dishpan Gardening

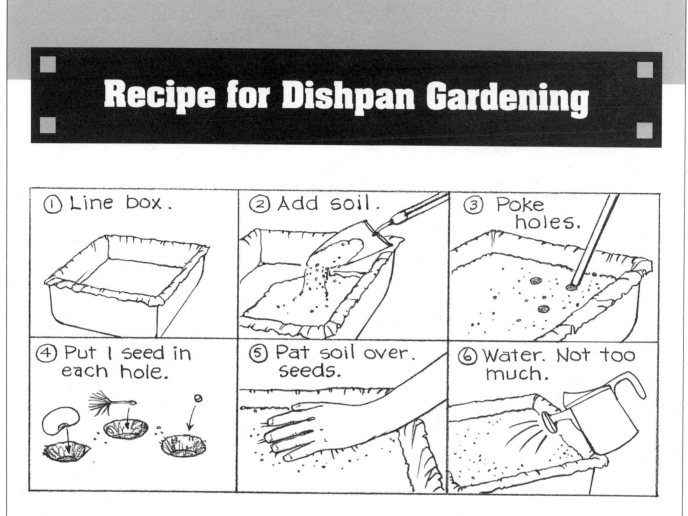

① Line box.

② Add soil.

③ Poke holes.

④ Put 1 seed in each hole.

⑤ Pat soil over seeds.

⑥ Water. Not too much.

Gardening Instructions

- Copy the garden recipe onto a large chart or onto individual cards.

- Talk about the pictures with small groups of children before they plant.

- While children make gardens, have them look at the pictures to see what they need to do.

- Help children talk about what they are doing.

- Optional:

  a. If children use plastic dishpans, do not have them line the box (step 1).

  b. Children can use a measuring stick to poke holes. Make a measuring stick by marking a straw, stick, or coffee stirrer 1/4" from one end. Tell children to make holes as deep as the mark.

  c. Place large-holed chicken wire on top of soil. Have the children plant only one seed in each wire space. This avoids over-crowding plants.

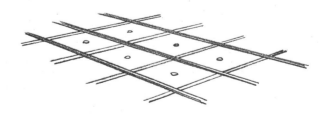

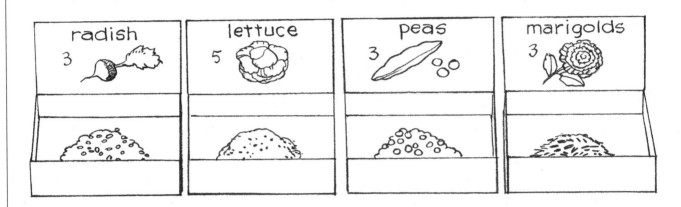

d. Allow children to choose their own seeds. Set up seeds so that children can see how many of each type to take. Provide a picture of what the seed will grow into.

Tip: Give children a piece of masking tape to stick seeds onto until they're ready to plant. They're easy to remove, and small seeds won't blow away or get lost.

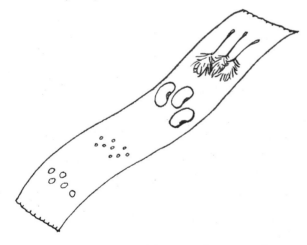

■ Encourage the children to observe and care for their own gardens.

Which Seeds to Plant

Look for seeds that complete a growth cycle quickly, or if school ends for the summer, plant seeds that can mature indoors or before summer comes. These seeds will mature in a very sunny window:

Burpee's Pixie Hybrid Tomato

Royal Oak leaf lettuce

sweet basil

garden cress (takes only 10 days)

bean sprouts

These seeds mature in a spring outdoor dishpan garden:

Cherry Belle radish (22 days)

French breakfast radish (23 days)

sweet early green peas (about 60 days)

loose head lettuces (Black Seeded Simpson, 45 days, Salad Bowl, 45 days)

Flowers that will grow in springtime outdoor gardens:

nasturtiums

marigolds

bachelor buttons (cornflower)

zinnia

Recipe for Chi Tong
(Chinese Chicken Soup)

CHI TONG 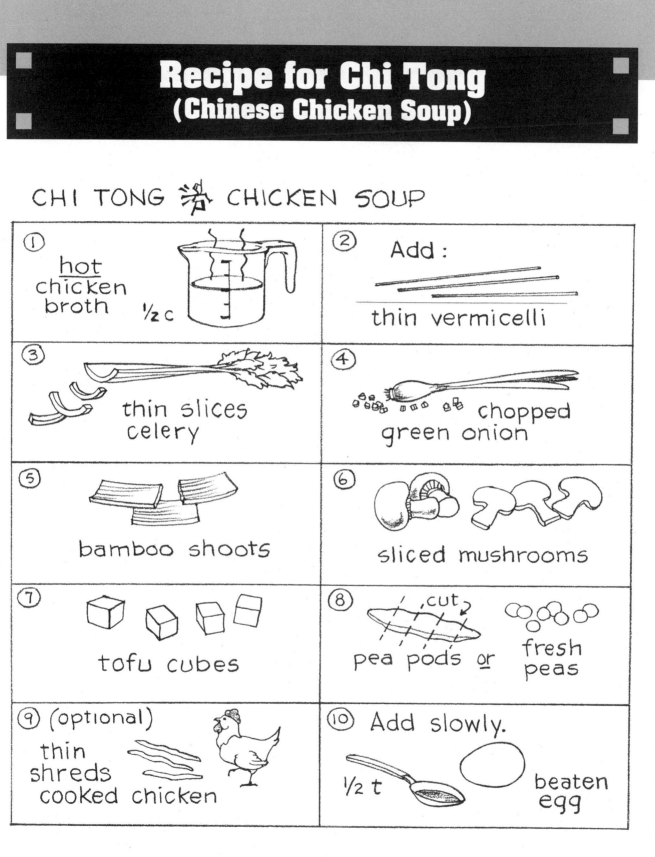 CHICKEN SOUP

① hot chicken broth ½ c

② Add : thin vermicelli

③ thin slices celery

④ chopped green onion

⑤ bamboo shoots

⑥ sliced mushrooms

⑦ tofu cubes

⑧ cut pea pods or fresh peas

⑨ (optional) thin shreds cooked chicken

⑩ Add slowly. ½ t beaten egg

from *Cook and Learn: A Child's Cook Book* by Beverly Veitch and Thelma Harms, published by Addison-Wesley Publishing Company.

Recipe for Cheese Pretzels

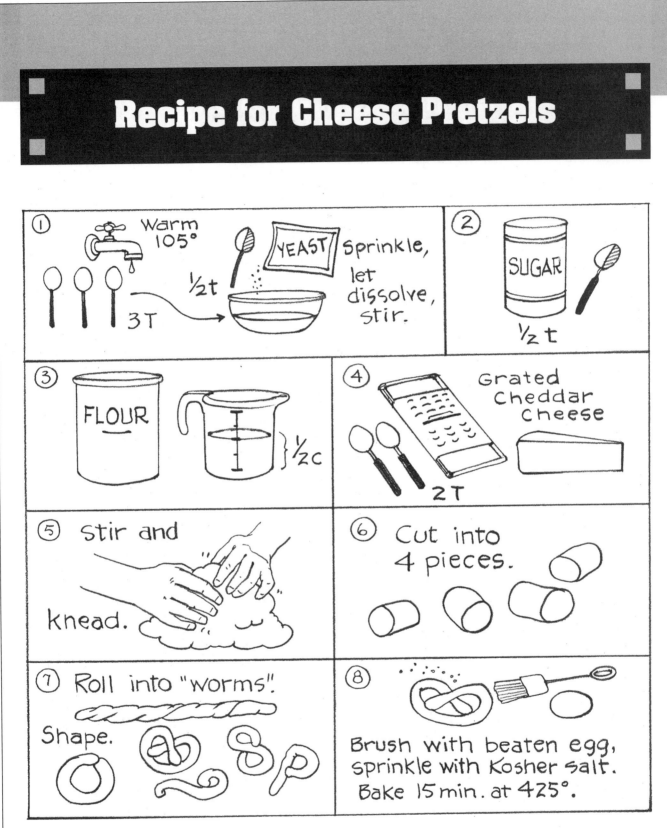

1. Warm 105° 3T ½t YEAST Sprinkle, let dissolve, stir.

2. SUGAR ½ t

3. FLOUR ½ c

4. Grated Cheddar Cheese 2T

5. Stir and knead.

6. Cut into 4 pieces.

7. Roll into "worms". Shape.

8. Brush with beaten egg, sprinkle with Kosher salt. Bake 15 min. at 425°.

from *Cook and Learn: A Child's Cook Book* by Beverly Veitch and Thelma Harms, published by Addison-Wesley Publishing Company.

Recipe for Stone Soup

1. Have each child bring in a vegetable that can go into the soup. Include potatoes, carrots, cabbage, green beans, onions, tomatoes.

2. Children can help wash vegetables, peel as needed, and cut up.

3. The vegetables can then be added to a large pot of chicken or beef broth or tomato juice (1/2 cup per child). Some barley can be added if you wish, as well as a little salt and pepper. Cook until the vegetables are soft.

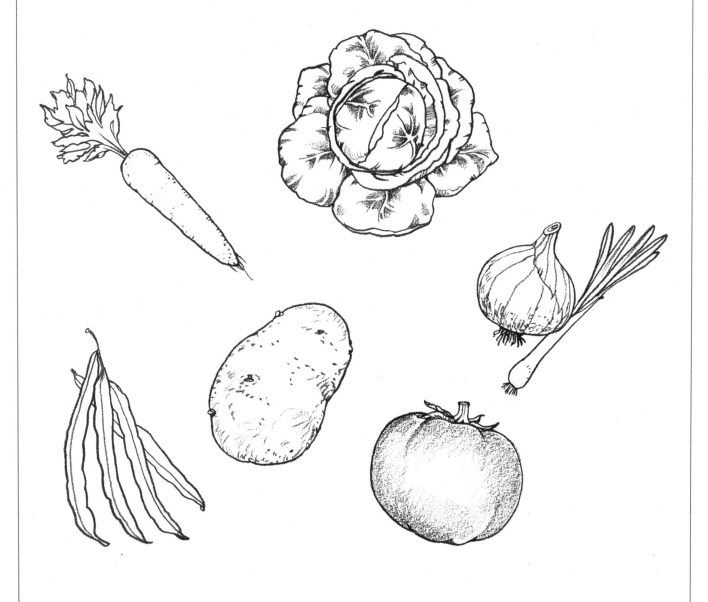

Recipe for Washing Hands

1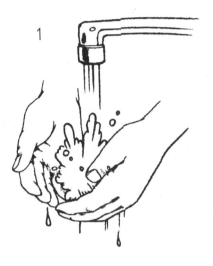

2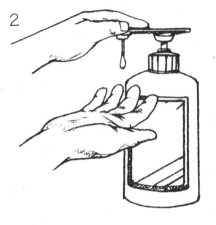

3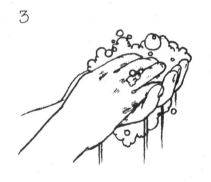

4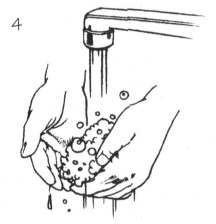

5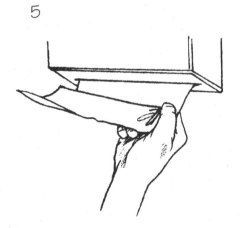

6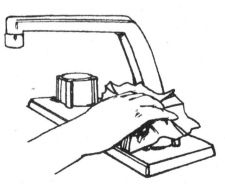

Appendix F: Recipes

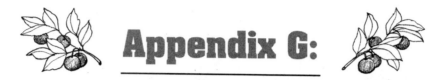

Appendix G:
Cookbooks to Use with Children

Cookbooks to Use with Children

Coats, Carolyn, and Pamela Smith. *Come Cook with Me! A Cookbook for Kids.* Orlando, FL: Carolyn Coats Bestsellers, 1989.

Easy and nutritious recipes for breakfast, lunch, snacks, and dinner. Includes a section on manners and table setting.

Copage, Eric V. *KWANZAA: An African-American Celebration of Culture and Cooking.* New York: William Morrow, 1991.

Proverbs and stories to illustrate the principles of Kwanzaa and recipes to help put together a Kwanzaa celebration. Includes highlights of African-American history.

Goodwin, Mary, and Gerry Pollen. *Creative Food Experiences for Children.* Washington, DC: Center for Science in the Public Interest, 1974.

This book offers a variety of recipes and food-learning activities that can be used with children to discover new ways of preparing different types of foods from the major food groups. It also includes basic nutrition education, the values of different food sources, and resource materials.

Klutz Press, Editors. *Kids Cooking: A Very Slightly Messy Manual.* Palo Alto, CA: Klutz Press, 1987.

Recipes that older children can prepare for themselves or that preschoolers can prepare with the help of an adult. Also includes directions for making play dough, face paint, and finger paints.

Marbach, Ellen, Martha Plass, and Lily O'Connell. *Nutrition in a Changing World: A Curriculum for Preschool.* Washington, DC: The Nutrition Foundation, Inc., 1979.

Preschool-kindergarten curriculum consisting of sequential units that include activities designed to be easily integrated into standard courses of studies, pre- and post-tests, background information, and lists of resource materials.

McClenahan, Pat, and Ida Jaqua. *Cool Cooking for Kids.* Belmont, CA: Fearon-Pitman, 1976.

This cookbook and curriculum guide can be used for teaching cooking and nutrition creatively. The book offers a collection of recipes that preschoolers can prepare and enjoy with or without using heat, plus various food-related activities.

Schlabach, Joetta Handrich. *Extending the Table: A World Community Cookbook.* Scottsdale, PA: Herald Press, 1991.

A Mennonite book of stories and recipes collected from around the world. Many recipes can be used in group cooking activities with preschoolers.

Veitch, Beverly, and Thelma Harms. *Cook and Learn: A Child's Cook Book.* Menlo Park, CA: Addison-Wesley, 1980.

Single-portion, picture-word recipes that all children can prepare for themselves are presented in sequenced steps; includes how to set up cooking experiences and why they are beneficial to children's learning. Many ethnic and nutritious recipes are included. Also available from the same publisher is the *Cook and Learn* teacher's guide, *Learning from Cooking Experiences* by Thelma Harms, designed for use with *Cook and Learn* but appropriate for use with any cooking experience; focuses on creation of a safe environment that encourages independence, reasoning, and oral expression.

Wannamaker, Nancy, Kristen Hearn, and Sherrill Richarz. *More Than Graham Crackers.* Washington, DC: National Association for the Education of Young Children, 1979.

A resource for teachers and parents that includes nutritious recipes from the four food groups and activities to extend each cooking experience, plus nutrition information and a resource list.

Williamson, Sarah, and Zachary Williamson. *Kids Cook: Fabulous Food for the Whole Family.* Charlotte, VT: Williamson Publishing, 1992.

A collection of recipes written by two children. Recipes are divided into three levels of difficulty. Includes suggestions for making recipes more nutritious.

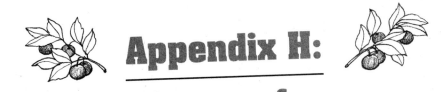

Appendix H:
Pictures for
Feeding Happy Tooth Activity

Pictures for
Feeding Happy Tooth Activity

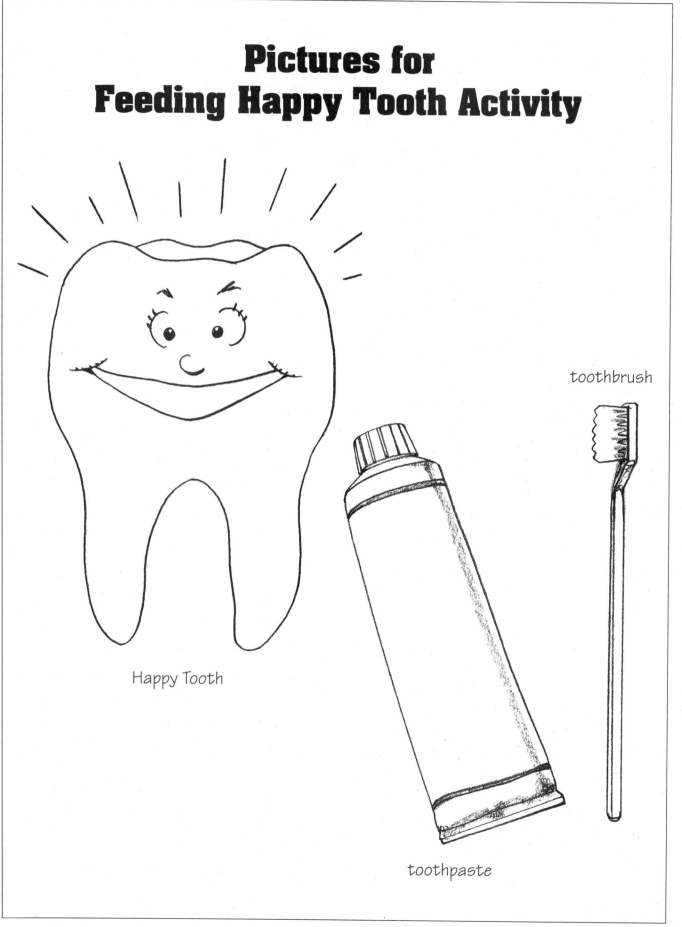

toothbrush

Happy Tooth

toothpaste

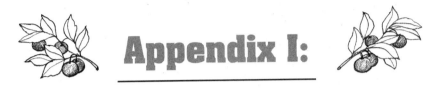

Appendix I:

Nursery Rhymes That Include Foods

Appendix I: Nursery Rhymes That Include Foods

Nursery Rhymes
That Include Foods

Peter, Peter, Pumpkin Eater

Peter, Peter Pumpkin Eater
Had a wife but couldn't keep her.
Put her in a pumpkin shell,
And there he kept her very well!

There Was an Old Woman Who Lived in a Shoe

There was an old woman who lived in a shoe,
She had so many children she didn't know what to do.
She gave them some broth without any bread
And kissed them all warmly
And put them to bed.

Little Miss Muffet

Little Miss Muffet
Sat on a tuffet
Eating her curds and whey.

Along came a spider
Who sat down beside her,
And frightened Miss Muffet away.

Little Jack Horner

Little Jack Horner
Sat in a corner
Eating his Christmas pie.

He stuck in his thumb,
And pulled out a plum,
And said, "What a good boy am I!"

This Little Piggie Went to Market

This little piggie went to market,
And this little piggie stayed home.
This little piggie ate roast beef,
And this little piggie had none.
And this little piggie cried Wee! Wee! Wee!
All the way home!

Old Mother Hubbard

Old Mother Hubbard
Went to the cupboard
To give her poor doggie a bone.

But when she got there,
The cupboard was bare,
So the poor little doggie got none.

Jack Sprat

Jack Sprat would eat no fat,
His wife would eat no lean.
And so between the two of them,
They licked the platter clean.

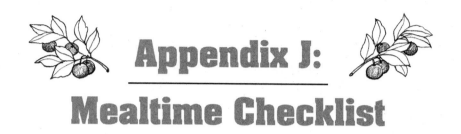

Appendix J:
Mealtime Checklist

Mealtime Checklist

This checklist was originally developed as part of the nutrition training resource, *Nutrition Education for Child Care*, by T. Harms, M. Farthing, S. Roholt, M. Clark, and D. Cryer, Division of Child Nutrition, North Carolina Department of Public Instruction.

Mealtime Checklist

This checklist will help you think about the setting for eating created for the children in your group. The checklist helps focus attention on the before-eating setting, during-eating setting, and after-eating setting.

Please think about these questions and answer them for your group. If you are working with others, discuss answers. After completing the checklist, think about any changes that are needed to improve the mealtimes. The checklist can be repeated to see if the changes have helped to improve the eating setting.

To score, count up all "Yes" responses. A high score is best, so look carefully at all "No" responses and plan for change.

Before Eating

yes no

☐ ☐ 1. Did the before-eating activity help to calm and quiet the children?

☐ ☐ 2. Are a few children sent to wash hands at a time?

☐ ☐ 3. Do all children wash hands?

☐ ☐ 4. Do children take some part in food preparation?

☐ ☐ 5. Do children take part in setting the table?

☐ ☐ 6. Is there an interesting before-eating activity that children enjoy?

yes no

☐ ☐ 7. Does the activity last until the meal is ready to eat?

☐ ☐ 8. If the meal is late, does the teacher avoid having the children wait by providing an interesting activity for them?

☐ ☐ 9. Do the adults introduce new foods children will be eating by showing the food, providing a small taste, talking about where the food comes from, and so on?

During Eating

Physical Setup

yes no

☐ ☐ 1. Do all children sit at a table while eating?

☐ ☐ 2. Do children eat with a small group of other children that is right for their age and ability and allows for conversation?

(3-year-olds: 4 or 5 children per table)

(4–5 year olds: 6 or 7 children per table)

☐ ☐ 3. Do children eat in a clean, light, cheerful room?

yes	no	

yes   no

4. If the children eat in a dining room with other classes, is the tone of the dining room pleasant, unpressured, and relaxed?

5. Are tables and chairs the correct size for the children so that their feet can rest flat on the floor, and arms can rest easily on the table?

Food

1. Is all of the food easy for children to manage? For example, are foods cut in small pieces and liquids served in small cups?

2. Are foods nutritious and appealing to children?

Food Service

1. Are provisions made for children to serve themselves? For example, are child-size pitchers, serving bowls, and utensils used?

2. Do children determine their own serving size?

3. Do children choose which foods they put on their plates?

4. Do children pour their own beverages?

5. May children have second helpings?

6. Do children serve their own second helpings?

Social Setup (Adults)

1. Is an adult sitting with the children at each table?

2. Do the adults eat the same meal as the children at the table?

3. Do adults act as good role models? (For example, do adults taste all foods served, observe general rules of cleanliness, maintain a pleasant attitude, eat well?)

4. Do adults avoid pressuring children to eat? For example, do adults avoid insisting on a clean plate, using dessert as reward, or withholding favorite foods?

yes   no

5. Do adults encourage, but not force children to try a very small taste of new or unpopular foods?

6. Are adults understanding and patient when teaching table manners to children?

7. Do adults show children how to clean up after accidents without being unpleasant? For example, does the adult patiently help the child learn to use a sponge or mop without blaming the child for the spill?

8. Do adults encourage children's conversation during eating?

9. Do adults help children talk about the following topics during meals?

- Ideas that interest children such as animals or super-heroes

- Things children do at home or school such as T.V. shows, family outings, activities

- Plans children have for the near future, such as field trips, holidays

- The foods being eaten, such as where they come from and details about taste, color, texture, smell, sound, and name

Social Setup (Children)

1. Do children talk with others sitting near them?

2. Are all children allowed to eat at their own speed without feeling pressured?

3. Can a child who finishes eating before the others leave the table and go to another activity? For example, is a child allowed to look at a book, go to brush teeth and wash hands, or get ready for nap?

Tone

1. Is the mealtime tone relaxed, pleasant, and interesting?

After Eating

yes	no		
☐	☐	1.	Do children have a role in clearing and cleaning the table after eating?
☐	☐	2.	Do all children rinse their mouths or brush their teeth and wash their hands?
☐	☐	3.	Are only a few children at a time sent to take care of hands and teeth?

yes	no		
☐	☐	4.	Is the next activity ready for children?
☐	☐	5.	Is the transition to the next activity unrushed and cheerful?

General Questions

yes	no		
☐	☐	1.	Looking back over the entire eating experience, did the teacher organize the before-, during-, and after-eating routine smoothly? What part of the routine can be improved? (Answer below.)
☐	☐	2.	Have the children been helped to be as independent as possible during the entire eating experience? What can be done to increase independence? (Answer below.)

yes	no		
☐	☐	3.	Is the setting convenient for adults and children? What can be improved in the physical or social setting? (Answer below.)
☐	☐	4.	Was the eating experience positive for both the children and the adults? What can be changed to improve the experience? (Answer below.)

Suggestions for improvement: _____

_____

_____

_____

_____

_____

_____

_____

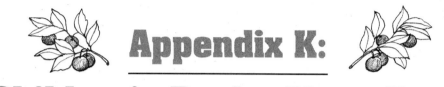

Appendix K:
Children's Books About Food

Children's Books About Food

About Baking and Bread

Asch, Frank. *Sand Cake.* New York: Parents Magazine Press, 1978.

Papa Bear uses his imagination to bake a delicious sand cake for Baby Bear and Mama Bear.

de Paola, Tomie. *Watch Out For the Chicken Feet in Your Soup.* New York: Prentice Hall (Simon & Schuster), 1974.

Joey and his friend Eugene visit Joey's grandmother. They eat a big lunch, and then Eugene gets to help make bread dolls.

Galdone, Paul. *The Gingerbread Boy.* Boston: Clarion Books (Houghton Mifflin), 1983.

In this traditional tale the gingerbread boy runs away to avoid being eaten.

———. *The Little Red Hen.* Boston: Clarion Books (Houghton Mifflin), 1983.

No one helps the little red hen do the work when she bakes a cake, so she eats the whole cake all by herself.

Morris, Ann. *Bread, Bread, Bread.* New York: Mulberry (William Morrow), 1993.

This richly illustrated book celebrates the many different uses and kinds of bread throughout the world.

Sendak, Maurice. *In the Night Kitchen.* New York: Harper & Row, 1970; paperback, New York: HarperCollins Children's Books, 1985.

A little boy dreams about bread being baked overnight by some funny bakers.

About Butter

Lindman, Maj. *Snipp, Snapp, Snurr and the Buttered Bread.* Cutchogue, NY: Buccaneer Books, 1993.

Milk must be gotten from a cow before butter can be churned.

About Eggs

San Souci, Robert D. *The Talking Eggs.* New York: Dial Books for Young Readers (Penguin USA), 1989.

Beautiful illustrations bring to life the story of magic stews and talking eggs.

Seuss, Dr. *Green Eggs and Ham.* New York: Random Books, 1960.

It turns out that green eggs and ham taste good, after all.

About Fish

Elkin, Benjamin. *Six Foolish Fishermen.* Chicago: Children's Press, 1986.

A small boy solves the foolish fishermen's problem and gets fish as a reward.

About Fruits and Vegetables

Aliki. *The Story of Johnny Appleseed.* Upper Saddle River, NJ: Prentice Hall, 1987.

Johnny Appleseed plants seeds that grow into trees.

Ehlert, Lois. *Eating the Alphabet: Fruits and Vegetables from A to Z.* Orlando, FL: Harcourt Brace Jovanovich, 1989.

An alphabet of common and uncommon fruits and vegetables, from apple to zucchini, including huckleberry, jicama, radicchio, and xigua, is beautifully illustrated.

Ginsburg, Mirra. *Mushroom in the Rain.* New York: Macmillan, 1990.

A mushroom grows bigger and bigger to provide shelter for animals in the rain.

Kimmelman, Leslie. *Frannie's Fruits.* New York: HarperCollins, 1989.

The author describes a day in the life of Frannie's fruit stand, which sells fruits, vegetables, and flowers on Highway 57.

Krauss, Ruth. *The Carrot Seed.* New York: Festival (HarperCollins Children's Books), 1993.

A tiny seed grows into a huge carrot.

Lionni, Leo. *The Biggest House in the World.* New York: Pantheon, 1968; paperback, New York: Knopf Books for Young Children, 1987.

A snail lives on and eats a cabbage while growing too large to move when the cabbage is gone.

McCloskey, Robert. *Blueberries for Sal.* New York: Viking Children's Books, 1948; paperback, New York: Puffin Books, 1993.

People and bears both enjoy a blueberry harvest.

Potter, Beatrix. *The Tale of Peter Rabbit.* New York: Puffin Books, 1992.

Peter raids a farmer's garden and almost gets caught.

Tresselt, Alvin. *Autumn Harvest.* New York: Lothrop, Lee & Shepard, 1951; paperback, New York: Mulberry (Morrow), 1990.

Apples, pears, pumpkins, corn, and grains are harvested.

Zolotow, Charlotte. *Mr. Rabbit and the Lovely Present.* New York: Trophy (HarperCollins Children's Books), 1977; paperback and cassette, Pine Plains, NY: Live Oak Media, 1987.

Apples, pears, and grapes make a wonderful gift for mothers.

About Grains and Seeds

Asch, Frank. *Popcorn.* New York: Parents Magazine Press, 1979.

Sam, the bear, invites his friends over for a Halloween party. They all bring popcorn.

Dooley, Norah. *Everybody Cooks Rice.* San Diego, CA: Carolrhoda Books, 1991.

Carrie searches from house to house to find her brother Anthony. Everywhere she goes they're cooking rice, and it's never the same dish.

Tresselt, Alvin. *Autumn Harvest.* New York: Lothrop, Lee & Shepard, 1951; paperback, New York: Mulberry (Morrow), 1990.

Corn, grain, and other foods are harvested.

About Honey

Berenstain, Stanley and Janice. *The Big Honey Hunt.* New York: Beginner (Random House), 1962.

Father Bear decides to show his son how to find honey.

Milne, A. A. *Winnie the Pooh.* New York: Puffin Books, 1992.

Pooh, the honey-loving bear, has adventures with his friends.

About Milk

Asch, Frank. *Milk and Cookies.* New York: Parents Magazine Press, 1982.

Baby bear has a nightmare and dreams that a dragon drinks all his milk and eats all his cookies.

About Pancakes

Carle, Eric. *Pancakes Pancakes.* Saxonville, MA: Picture Book Studios, 1991.

> Pancakes are made from raw ingredients.

Sawyer, Ruth. *Journey Cake Ho.* New York: Puffin Books, 1978.

> A pancake rolls away to avoid being eaten.

About Soup

Brown, Marcia. *Stone Soup.* New York: Aladdin (Macmillan Children's Book Group), 1986.

> Three soldiers and the peasants of a village share and cooperate to make a wonderful vegetable beef soup for all to enjoy.

Sendak, Maurice. *Chicken Soup with Rice.* New York: HarperCollins Children's Books, 1962.

> Poems about the months, including a month in which it is nice to eat chicken soup with rice.

About Pleasant Eating Experiences in a Variety of Cultures

Bang, Molly. *The Paper Crane.* New York: Mulberry (William Morrow), 1987.

> An old man visits a poor restaurant. He pays for his dinner by leaving a paper crane that comes alive and dances.

Burden-Patmon, Denise. *Imani's Gift at Kwanzaa.* New York: Simon & Schuster, 1993.

> A young girl and her family learn the true meaning of Kwanzaa as they prepare for the evening feast.

Caines, Jeannette F. *Just Us Women.* New York: HarperCollins Children's Books, 1984.

> A young girl and her aunt travel to North Carolina, eating all the way.

Copage, Eric V. *KWANZAA: An African-American Celebration of Culture and Cooking.* New York: William Morrow, 1991.

> A book of stories and recipes for the celebration of Kwanzaa. The seven principles of Kwanzaa are emphasized throughout the book.

The National Council of Negro Women, Inc. *The Black Family Reunion Cookbook.* Memphis, TN: The Willmer Companies, 1991.

> Members of the National Council of Negro Women, Inc., share recipes and memories.

General Books About Cooking, Other Kitchen Activities, and Eating

Allison, Linda, and Martha Weston. *Eenie Meenie and Miney Math! Math Play for You and Your Preschooler.* Covelo, CA: Little Yolla Bolly Press, 1993.

> The authors suggest short and simple ideas for introducing your child to math using daily routines and events. Kitchen activities are included.

Carle, Eric. *Today Is Monday.* New York: Philomel Books (Putnam Publishing Group), 1993.

> Eric Carle offers a vibrant rendition of a familiar children's song. Children will love filling in the foods as they repeat the food for each day of the week.

———. *The Very Hungry Caterpillar.* New York: Putnam, 1986.

> A very hungry caterpillar eats his way through this story.

Hoban, Russell. *Bread and Jam for Frances.* New York: Scholastic, 1964.

> Frances learns that there are more good things to eat than bread and jam.

Kraus, Robert. *Leo the Late Bloomer.* New York: Harper Collins Children's Books, 1971.

Leo, a sloppy-eating lion cub, grows into a neat-eating young lion.

Rey, Margaret, and Alan J. Shallek. *Curious George Goes to a Restaurant.* Boston: Houghton Mifflin, 1988.

Curious George the monkey goes to a restaurant with the man in the yellow hat. George makes a big mess and then saves the day.

Slepian, Jan, and Ann Seidler. *The Hungry Thing.* New York: Scholastic, 1988.

Grownups can't understand Hungry Thing when he asks for food to eat. A little boy guesses what he's really asking for.

———. *The Hungry Thing Returns.* New York: Scholastic, 1993.

The Hungry Thing and Small Hungry Thing visit a school. They talk in mixed up rhymes. See if the children can figure out what they want before you tell them.

———. *The Hungry Thing Goes to a Restaurant.* New York: Scholastic, 1993.

The Hungry Thing visits a restaurant. When he asks for papple moose, the waiters try to guess what he really wants to eat.

Vincent, Gabrielle. *Ernest and Celestine's Picnic.* New York: Mulberry (William Morrow), 1988.

Ernest the bear and Celestine the mouse plan a picnic. Even rain can't dampen their spirits.

About Recycling

Gibbons, Gail. *Recycle! A Handbook for Kids.* Boston: Little, Brown, 1992.

Children learn how they can make recycling a habit.

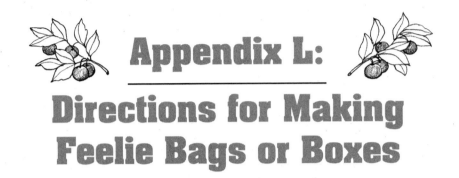

Appendix L:

Directions for Making Feelie Bags or Boxes

Directions for Making Feelie Bags or Boxes

Feelie Bag

1. Place a plastic container inside a large, stretchy sock. You might use a clean yogurt container or a plastic food storage container.

2. Place something in the container that is safe for the child to feel.

3. Show the child how to reach inside the sock and touch the thing in the container without pulling it out.

4. Let the children guess what they are feeling.

Feelie Box

1. Cut a 3- to 4-inch hole in the end of a large shoe box.

2. Tape or glue a piece of material on the inside of the box so that it covers the hole like a curtain.

3. Place something in the box that is safe for the child to feel.

4. Put the cover on the box.

5. Show the child how to reach inside and touch the thing in the box without pulling it out.

6. Let children guess what they are feeling.

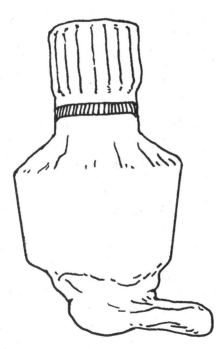

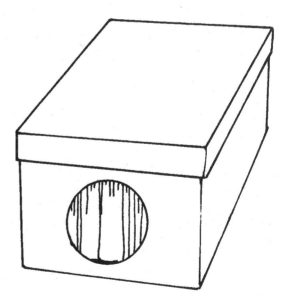

Training Manual for
Nutrition Activities
for Preschoolers

Contents

Introduction

This training manual provides a variety of activities for introducing early childhood educators to the resource book, *Nutrition Activities for Preschoolers*. The activities can be used for large or small group sessions or can be used more informally by individuals.

Trainers need to be aware that what we eat has deep ties to home, family, and culture. It can, therefore, be an emotionally laden subject and needs to be handled with respect for individual preferences and sensitivity to the many differences that exist in our country.

Goals of training

Learning to use *Nutrition Activities for Preschoolers* will help you achieve the following goals:

- To review nutrition information about young children to help you serve healthful foods that meet their nutritional needs

- To consider ways to make meals and snacks pleasant experiences that encourage children to enjoy healthful foods

- To integrate nutrition activities into the regular daily program in all types of early childhood settings

Preparing yourself as a trainer

Trainers conducting this workshop will undoubtedly come from a variety of backgrounds. Some trainers will come from nutrition- and health-related fields; others from early childhood development and education-related fields. A working knowledge of both nutrition and early childhood education is needed to effectively guide a group of participants learning to use nutrition activities. *Nutrition Activities for Preschoolers* gives practical, basic information on both subjects. Read the book carefully before organizing a training session.

If the trainer will be required to teach early childhood staff from a variety of programs, it is wise to have some firsthand experience with the different types of settings and know something about their unique characteristics. For example:

- How do part-day preschools and childcare centers differ and what are their similarities?

- How do family childcare homes provide early childhood activities in a home setting?

- What are the pluses and minuses for a childcare center of having food delivered versus preparing it on site?

The participants in the training will have a lot to say about their children and their settings. The trainers can make good use of this wealth of information and experience by encouraging discussion and sharing throughout the training session.

Handling different preschool settings

Since there are many different types of preschool settings, try to include several people from similar settings in a group so that no one feels isolated. For example, a preschool teacher may feel out of place in a group of family childcare providers because the settings are so different, whereas several preschool teachers can share information more confidently with the group pointing out similarities and differences in preschool.

Be prepared to address similarities and differences in settings, keeping in mind that the activities in *Nutrition Activities for Preschoolers* are equally suitable for use in all early childhood settings, including family childcare, childcare centers, Head Start, kindergartens, and part- or full-day preschool programs. Individual variation in program content, space, and equipment will, of course, determine which activities are easier or more difficult to implement.

Adapting for individual children

Children of widely differing abilities and from diverse backgrounds attend early childhood programs together. As with all other aspects of the program, the teacher will need to select the nutrition activities that best suit the children's needs. Each of the activities in *Nutrition Activities for Preschoolers* is described clearly, including what materials are needed, how to set up so children can participate independently, and what the teacher can say to help children learn more from their play. Each activity has several suggestions for ways to extend themes, tasks, and objectives.

As a teacher looks through the book, the level of abstract thinking required for each activity will become apparent. There is also a recommended age level noted on each activity, which can be used as a general guideline to determine level of difficulty. It should be emphasized that the activities are suggestions; teachers are free to adapt, change, and create new activities as they implement the hands-on activity ideas.

Encouraging active participation

Your training session should encourage active participation through discussion, clarification, and trying out selected activities to see how they work. The participants need to experience some of the hands-on nutrition activities themselves during the training in order to learn how to present the activities to children.

Keep lecturing to a minimum. Consider yourself to be an active discussion leader who can underline important points, encourage sharing, and summarize effectively. Practice what you preach by providing healthful snacks for the participants during the training. Serve fruit and fruit juices, crisp vegetable slices, breads, crackers, and spreads low in fat, salt, and sugar.

Planning training sessions

When you plan a training session, take the following into consideration:

1. *How will the participants be using the training?*

   Some training sessions will be held for trainers such as community college instructors, childcare consultants, and Department of Public Education staff, who will in turn conduct training for teachers of young children. Other training sessions will be held for teachers of young children. The sessions for trainers need to include a discussion of appropriate techniques for training adults and suggestions for planning workshops, as well as specific training activities to use in the sessions.

   Teachers who will be working with children may be most interested in discovering ways to solve meal and snack problems and ideas for adding nutrition activities to various learning centers and meal and snack times. General content issues relating to presenting nutrition facts, creating pleasant mealtimes, setting up activity centers, and providing nutrition activities as part of the ongoing classroom should be covered with both groups.

2. *How long will the training session last?*

   Length of training can vary from a short session of one to three hours, to longer sessions lasting a whole day or even several days.

3. *What is the basic training content?*

   Regardless of the length of the training session, each part of *Nutrition Activities for Preschoolers* should be introduced. The participants can, at a minimum, turn to selected pages in the book to see how the five steps to successful nutrition education are handled. Make sure to show how the nutrition activities are organized to fit easily into everyday meal and snack times and learning centers. The newsletters and other appendix materials should also be introduced.

   In each training session, no matter how short, include at least one of the Optional Participation Activities—a discussion, role-playing exercise, or a hands-on activity. In longer sessions, more hands-on activities can be included.

4. *What training materials are needed?*

   It is best for each participant to have a copy of *Nutrition Activities for Preschoolers* to use during the training, though transparencies of specific pages referred to throughout the "Suggested Training Content" can be used instead. For group training sessions, overhead transparencies of some of the graphics may be helpful even if each participant has the book. Suggestions for graphics that can be used for transparencies are given in specific training activities. Additional equipment or supplies may be required for specific nutrition activities.

5. *How can the content be presented in an interesting, nonthreatening way?*

Throughout the training session it is essential for the group leader to be respectful of and sensitive to the participants' ideas and feelings. As participants share their own experiences and their attitudes toward children's nutrition, their nutrition habits and preferences will become apparent. Cultural and personal differences may emerge. It is the group leader's job to teach the nutritional information that will help shape children's healthful eating habits and to introduce the activities for use in the classroom in a nonjudgmental way.

Suggested training content

The following training sequence can be modified to meet the needs of participants:

I.   Introduction to the group

Activity: Help participants become acquainted with one another as you get to know who is in the group. Have each person give a brief introduction and find out the following information:

- Who are the members of the group?
- What types of programs for preschoolers do they work with?
- What age groups do they have, and are there any children with disabilities in their groups?
- What meals and snacks do they serve?
- Is there anything in particular they want to be sure to learn?

In a very short session with larger groups, individual introductions may not be possible, but the group leader should at least determine types of programs, age groups, and special concerns.

Activity: If the training will be several hours long, go through an agenda with the participants. Let them know the schedule that will be followed, including information about meals or snacks and breaks. Provide an overview of how the training will proceed and briefly explain the content and training.

II. Introduction to the book
Nutrition Activities for Preschoolers

Activity: Introduce the idea that nutrition education involves more than just serving healthful foods or doing a short-term nutrition unit with preschoolers. Then briefly introduce the Five Steps to Successful Nutrition Education on page 2 of *Nutrition Activities for Preschoolers.*

Be sure to cover the following points:

■ Step 1 gives nutritional information to help select, prepare, and serve appropriate amounts of healthful foods to children.

■ Steps 2, 3, and 4 address the need for pleasant mealtimes to establish good attitudes toward food.

■ Step 5 suggests ways to provide nutrition activities in the various learning centers of a preschool setting, as well as during meals and snacks.

Activities for Step 1:
Serve healthful foods

Activity: Review the 20 Nutrition Facts to Think About (pages 4–8). Either use transparencies that you can project using an overhead projector or have the participants look at their books for the 20 Nutrition Facts.

Be sure to cover the following points:

■ Facts 1–8 focus on meeting children's nutritional needs.

■ Facts 9–14 focus on respecting children's foods choices.

■ Facts 15–20 focus on encouraging children to enjoy healthful foods.

Activity: Review basic information about how to meet children's nutritional needs. (Transparencies of all pages suggested here would be helpful.)

Be sure to cover the following points:

■ Explain the relative amounts of different foods needed in a healthful diet. Use the six basic foods group chart on page 10, the Food Guide Pyramid on page 11, and "Suggested Servings for Preschoolers" on page 12.

■ Children should never be forced to eat food they do not like. Comparable foods can be substituted (See page 14 and Appendix A for food substitutes.)

■ Adults should ensure that there is enough iron in the foods served to children. Use the graphic on page 18 ("Serve Foods High in Iron") to illustrate Nutrition Fact 6.

■ Foods that encourage good health should be served frequently. Use the graphics on pages 16 and 17 ("Do Children a Favor") to discuss the substitution of more healthful foods for less healthful ones.

Optional Participation Activities

1. Reading food container labels

   Bring in a number of labels from food containers. Include labels for comparison of nutritional content, such as labels from tuna packed in oil and tuna packed in water, dry cereals with and without added salt and sugar, regular and reduced fat mayonnaise or margarine. Have enough labels to distribute so that several small groups of participants can work. Provide measuring spoons and measuring cups so that participants can see how much of a particular food makes up the serving size indicated on the label. Have each small group report back to the whole group.

   Have participants look at all the labels and find out which foods are highest in calories, fat, vitamins, and minerals. Ask them to look at the ingredients labels to find out the contents of the foods. Remind participants that the ingredients are listed in descending order from most to least.

2. Foods with child appeal

   Using nutrition facts 10 and 18, have the participants suggest some foods that have child appeal. Discuss what properties give foods child appeal.

3. Planning nutritious snacks

   Using the Food Guide Pyramid and the Suggested Servings Chart, have participants plan nutritious snacks that they could get the ingredients for, prepare, and serve in their settings, and that their children might enjoy.

Activities for Step 2:
Provide pleasant meal and snack times

Activity: Review nutrition facts 11, 12, 14, 18, 19, and 20, which are most closely related to pleasant mealtimes.

Be sure to cover the following points:

■ Avoid having children wait in a group before meals or snacks by providing a short period of quiet play, such as listening to a story or singing.

■ Have each child wash his or her hands thoroughly.

■ Have a few children help with setting the tables.

- Provide child-sized serving utensils.

- Have an adult sit with the children to encourage pleasant meal-time conversation and set an example for good manners and healthful eating habits rather than act as a police officer.

- Never use food as a reward or punishment.

- Encourage independence in cleanup; do not hurry slow eaters; have a smooth transition to the next activity.

- Point out the Mealtime Checklist in Appendix J and discuss how participants might use it.

Activity: Have the group discuss what makes a pleasant mealtime for them as adults. What makes a meal a pleasant, social experience? Use the characteristics that the group suggests to generate a list and record it on the chalkboard or on chart paper so that everyone can see it. Then have the group apply the characteristics to their early childhood setting. Discuss what they would need to change to make mealtimes more pleasant in their early childhood setting.

Optional Participation Activities

1. Finding solutions to ensure pleasant meals and snacks

   In small groups, have participants describe problems they have that keep snack or mealtimes from being pleasant in their settings. Have each group report back to the whole group, and let the whole group suggest solutions for the most common problems.

2. Handling sanitation and safety

   In small groups, discuss how to best handle the sanitation and the safety aspects of pleasant mealtimes. Health considerations include hand washing and other sanitation procedures. Safety includes making sure children do not choke while eating. After the group generates ideas, use the book to point out handwashing (page 23) and the Practicing Handwashing activity (page 52); children cleaning up after themselves (page 25); choking hazards (page 19).

3. Planning for pleasant times before, during, and after meals or snacks

   Discuss what can be done before mealtimes, during mealtimes, and after mealtimes to make them pleasant for the children. Pay special attention to ways in which participants have been successful at handling children individually or in small groups rather than as a large group. Remind the participants that developing independence and learning to get along with one another help make meals good learning experiences as well as pleasant social experiences. After the discussion, have the participants review pages 22–28 for additional ideas.

Point out the Mealtime Checklist in Appendix J and have participants complete the checklist for their own classroom or for a familiar program.

Activities for Step 3:
Work with parents to encourage healthful eating habits

Activity: Review commonly used forms of teacher-parent communication, such as posting menus and talking with parents at drop-off and pick-up times.

Be sure to cover the following points:

- Regular communication between parents and teachers is essential.
- Respect for parents' values must be communicated even when parents' ideas differ from the teacher's.

Activity: Discuss with the participants what sort of information they need from parents and what sort of information they feel parents need from them. Refer participants to pages 30–34 of the book.

Activity: Show the participants the newsletters available in Appendix B on *Nutrition Activities for Preschoolers*. Discuss how they might use the newsletters.

Activity: Discuss with the participants how they can bring cultural differences into the program in a positive way. Ask what their experience has been in this area. Refer participants to page 34 of the book.

Optional Participation Activities

1. Planning for communication with parents

   Break into small groups. Have each group make a plan for providing parents with nutrition information (page 31). Ask group members to be sure to consider what would be possible in their own settings. Have the small groups report back to the whole group.

2. Role-play a parent-teacher conversation about nutrition.

   Situation A: A parent is going to bring a treat to celebrate her child's birthday. The teacher wants to start to serve healthful party foods. How does she communicate this to the parent without being offensive? What suggestions can she offer?

Situation B: There is one family in the program who wants their child to be on a very low-calorie diet to prevent the possibility of the child becoming overweight. They insist that their child be served limited amounts of foods that are low in calories. The child seems tired and fragile, and you are concerned about the adequacy of his diet.

- Role-play a consultation with a pediatrician or nutritionist if nutrition is not the participant's area of expertise.

- Role-play a meeting to discuss the issue with the parent.

Activity: Discuss the importance of having the teacher sit and eat with the children at meal and snack times.

Be sure to cover the following points:

- The teacher should eat the same meal the children eat.

- The teacher's actions speak louder than words. The children need to see the teacher eating healthful meals and snacks.

Optional Participation Activities

1. Childhood memories

   Discuss early food memories. What did our families consider healthful foods? Have our ideas changed? If so, how? How have our food preferences changed over time?

2. Food diaries

   Have each participant make out a food intake diary for the day before, including the foods eaten at breakfast, lunch, dinner, and snacks. Using the Food Guide Pyramid, have each person evaluate her or his food intake diary. This diary is completed from memory and may not be accurate, but the intent is for each participant to become aware of eating habits. This evaluation can also be made using the foods that the participants remember the children were served the day before.

3. Solutions to problems that prevent eating with children

   In small groups, discuss what keeps teachers from sitting down and eating meals and snacks with the children. Have each group generate a problems list. Then have the whole group suggest solutions.

Activities for Step 5:
Make nutrition activities part of the daily learning environment

Activity: Discuss the basics required for implementing nutrition education activities with preschoolers.

Be sure to cover the following points:

- Nutrition activities cannot be successfully integrated if the setting does not accommodate developmentally appropriate activities.

- Preschool settings should help children learn to communicate, to get along with others, to develop a positive self image, to develop gross- and fine-motor skills, and to develop basic learning and thinking skills.

- Preschool environments should be organized into learning centers that children can use daily during long periods of free play time. These centers should have many materials to use, convenient and accessible storage, and space to play.

- Learning centers should be organized so that children can be as independent as possible. (See page 42, Tips on Setting Up Learning Centers.)

- The daily schedule should make a variety of routines and activities possible with smooth, gradual transitions. (See page 44, Sample Schedule.)

Activity: Discuss the general guidelines that should be kept in mind when adding nutrition activities to a preschool environment. Go over the general guidelines on page 45, pointing out particularly talking with children, repeating nutrition facts, avoiding quizzing and pressure, and avoiding boring the children with unnecessary repetition or long explanations.

Optional Participation Activity

1. Problems in applying the learning center concept

   Conduct a short session with the whole group to identify problems in applying the learning center concept. Generate a problems list (space for only a few centers, lack of materials, wide age range with few preschoolers, and so on). Organize small groups to discuss particular problems and suggest solutions.

III. Practice with the nutrition activity ideas

Activity: Point out that the main section of *Nutrition Activities for Preschoolers* presents nutrition activities that can be done at meal and snack times and in the different learning centers.

Be sure to cover the following points:

- There are activities for Meal and Snack Time, the Art Center, Block Center, Book Center, Games Center, Music Center, Pretend Play Center, and Science and Math Center.

- All of the activities follow the same format.

- Each activity is related to a general area of nutrition education (Information for Good Food Choices, Encouraging Independence, Making Mealtimes Pleasant, Learning About Different Cultures, or Making Snacks for Parents).

- An appropriate age indication is given for each activity. Because preschoolers' developmental levels differ, deciding which activities are appropriate for individual children is, of course, left up to the discretion of the teacher.

Optional Participation Activities

In order to familiarize participants with the variety of activities designed for the different learning centers, two activities from each learning center and two from the meal and snack time have been chosen for participants to try.

   The Nutrition Activities are divided into eight sections. Depending on the number of people in your group, divide the total group into teams of two or more people. Give each team a choice of activities to try out and discuss.

   Below are suggestions for activities that can be used. You may also have some favorites that you want participants to try. In short training sessions, have the whole group do at least one activity.

1. Adding Nutrition Activities to Meal and Snack Times

   Practicing Handwashing (page 52)

   Follow the instructions. Find the handwashing steps in Appendix F.

   Discuss the following point:

   - How could you make this activity work in your setting?

   Recycling to Save Resources (page 58)

   Read the activity and extensions.

   Discuss the following points:

   - What could you recycle in your setting?

   - What recycled items can be used in art projects or put to other uses?

   - How would you explain recycling to the children?

2. Adding Nutrition Activities to the Art Center

Placemat Art (page 64)

Discuss the placemat activity and its extensions.
If there is time, let the participants make a placemat.

Discuss the following points:

- Would the children in the participants' groups be able to do this activity?
- What other things could the placemats be used for?

Making Favorite Foods Collage (page 66)

Bring in magazines participants can use to cut out food pictures. Include women's magazines, health magazines, weekly grocery advertisements, etc. to add to the variety. Let the participants make collages.

Discuss the following points:

- How could this activity be used in their settings?
- Would the extensions work?

3. Adding Nutrition Activities to the Block Center

Feeding Toy Animals (page 69)

Read the activity and the extension.

Discuss the following points:

- What additional foods are enjoyed by both animals and humans?
- If participants have live animals in the setting, how could they add to this activity?

Grocery Store Block Play (page 72)

Read the activity and the extensions carefully. Then have participants plan some activities to help children understand how and why things are stacked in the supermarket. For example, you might suggest that teachers show the children a picture of cans and containers on shelves and talk about how things are grouped together. Refer teachers to the "Pretending with Empty Food Containers" activity in the Pretend Play section and point out how the children might also stack empty food containers to make a store before doing the block activity.

Discuss the following points:

- Would taking a trip to the supermarket give the children more information to work with?
- How can you add information on size, shape, or number to this activity?

Nutrition Activities for Preschoolers

4. Adding Nutrition Activities to the Book Center

What We Ate for Breakfast Book (page 79)

Have paper and felt pens ready for the participants to make a book about what they ate for breakfast. Discuss the activity and extensions with a view to how to make them work best in the classroom.

Read and Make Soup (page 83)

Bring in some of the children's cookbooks listed in Appendix G. Have the participants read the activity and find some soup recipes.

Discuss the following point:

- Which of the extensions would work in their classrooms?

5. Adding Nutrition Activities to the Games Center

Food Containers Matching Game (page 92)

Read the activity and extensions carefully.

Discuss the following points:

- Would the activity work in their classroom?
- What food containers would they use with the children?

How Foods Help Us Matching Games (pages 179–187)

Read the activity and extension carefully, and locate the pictures for the activity in Appendix D.

Discuss the following points:

- Would this activity work with their children?
- How would they approach the game?
- How could they involve parents in making games?

6. Adding Nutrition Activities to the Music Center

Select one of the three variations on the songs in the Music section of the book. Try singing the song with the participants.

Discuss the following points:

- Is the song easy to learn and sing?
- Would their children like it?

7. Adding Nutrition Activities to the Pretend Play Center

Pretending with Empty Food Containers (pages 109–110)

Read the activity and extension carefully.

Discuss the following points:

- Would this activity work with their group?
- What are some ways to involve the parents in this activity?
- How could you find food containers that represent various cultures?
- How can you make the children aware of the different types of foods from many cultures?

Pretend Play About Foods That Do Not Come from the Supermarket (page 112)

Read the activity and extensions carefully.

Discuss the following points:

- What books could they read to the children to go with this activity?
- What are some additional foods people raise?

8. Adding Nutrition Activities to the Science and Math Center

Food Group Tasting Activities (page 120)

Using the Food Guide Pyramid, plan a series of food-tasting activities.

Discuss the following point:

- What other activities in the book could be used to help children understand how foods help keep us healthy? Look through the other activities to see which are most helpful.

Discovering Seeds in Fruits and Vegetables (page 123)

Bring in fruits and vegetables so that the participants can see their seeds. Have a good magnifying glass handy. Let them taste the fruits and vegetables also. Try some of the extensions suggested. Discuss the differences in the seeds.

Read the activity and extensions.

Discuss the following points:

- What are some fruits and vegetables that have interesting seeds for children to explore?
- What seeds are best to use for making comparisons?

Training Content Checklist

Final check before conducting training

In order to make sure that the participants are introduced to all of the sections of *Nutrition Activities for Preschoolers*, check off each item as you include it in your training:

- [ ] The 20 Nutrition Facts
- [ ] The Food Guide Pyramid
- [ ] Suggested Serving Sizes Chart
- [ ] Respecting Children's Likes and Dislikes
- [ ] Practicalities of Providing Pleasant Meals and Snacks
- [ ] Ideas for Providing Information and Resources for Parents
- [ ] Basic Information on Learning Centers
- [ ] Nutrition Activities to Add to Learning Centers
- [ ] Newsletters for Parents
- [ ] Pieces, Patterns, and Recipes for Games and Activities
- [ ] Checklist to Observe Mealtimes
- [ ] Children's Booklist
- [ ] Children's Cookbooks
- [ ] Nursery Rhymes about Foods
- [ ] Foods to Substitute

During the training session make sure that

- [ ] The participants get to ask questions, look at the book, and discuss hands-on activities.
- [ ] The participants are given enough of an introduction to feel comfortable with the book and to be motivated to use it.
- [ ] The participants are shown that the activities can be used in all types of settings for preschoolers.
- [ ] The participants are shown that activities of varying difficulty are suitable for children of varying abilities.
- [ ] The participants are shown that the activities can be tailored to fit the needs of individual children and families.